Dr. Cass Ingram

Natural Cures *for* High Blood Pressure

D1115546

KNOWLEDGE HOUSE PUBLISHERS
Buffalo Grove, Illinois

First Edition

Printed in the United States of America

ISBN: 1-931078-14-9

Disclaimer: This book is not intended as a substitute for medical diagnosis or treatment. Anyone who has a serious disease should consult a physician before initiating any change in treatment or before beginning any new treatment.

To order this or additional Knowledge House books call 1-800-243-5242.

For book information visit: www.knowledgehousepublishers.com

For product information visit: www.oreganol.com

Contents

Introduction

Globally, high blood pressure is one of the most common conditions afflicting human beings. Medically, this condition is known as hypertension. Physicians claim to treat it successfully, that is with medication. In this book the terms high blood pressure and hypertension will be used interchangeably.

There is normal blood pressure, about 120/80. This is a measurement taken by a pressure sensitive device, which is wrapped around the arm. The pressure is a reflection of the pumping action of the heart against the arteries. It is the arterial tone, that is the muscular reaction of the arteries against the movement of blood within them, that results in the reading. The measurement is detecting pressure within the arteries originating from the heart, which is the pump. The normal range is well established, but levels from 110/70, which is, in fact, ideal, to 130/90 are accepted within the normal range. However, any deviation from this is regarded as abnormal.

In his book, *The Complete Guide to Living with High Blood Pressure*, Michael K. Rees, M.D. proclaims that high blood pressure should always be treated. However, his suggestions for treatment are purely medical, that is the use of potent drugs to lower blood pressure. This is never the premise of this book. Rather, the objective is that the cause of this condition must be treated. Yet, notice the key words in the title of Dr. Rees' book: *Living with it*. This is a disastrous attitude because high blood pressure is due to specific causes. It is these causes which must be determined and treated, so that the disease can be cured. Obviously, addressing the symptoms alone will fail to cure the disease.

In my medical training I observed numerous catastrophes, including stroke and sudden death, as a result of forcibly reducing the blood pressure. Yet, that is the method of treatment of which Dr. Rees writes. The fact is if a deliberate effort had been made to determine the exact cause in these cases the catastrophes could have been avoided. In other words, the patients could have survived or avoided permanent harm.

Doctors believe that high blood pressure is the disease. Yet, it cannot be so, because it is merely a symptom of an underlying condition. There is always a cause for high blood pressure. The secret is to determine the causes and treat it. Today, in high blood pressure patients this is rarely if ever achieved. The great error of the medical profession is, in fact, the neglect to determine the cause.

The purpose of this book is the discovery of the true causes of high blood pressure as well as various forms of heart disease. Here, the medical literature is reviewed, with emphasis on the pathology, that is the medical features, linked to these conditions. The benefit of this approach is that with the real cause identified the ideal treatment can be prescribed.

The fact is, the treatment for heart disease and high blood pressure is similar, because the causes are similar. This is true of the entire gamut of circulatory diseases, including hypertension, mitral valve prolapse, heart failure, hardening of the arteries, and coronary artery disease. Thus, this book is a thorough primer on the causes and cures for America's number one killer: circulatory diseases.

How the blood system operates

Without the blood pressure mechanism life would be impossible. The importance of this mechanism is demonstrated by simple facts. The human body is under the pressure of gravity. Yet, despite standing and sitting positions, both of which are against gravity, the blood circulates.The blood is able to move fully against gravity. Ultimately, it reaches the brain, as well as the rest of the body, often moving uphill. It is the pressure that develops within the bloodstream that allows this. The circulatory system is a closed loop; the heart is the pump. The pumping actions of the heart create pressure, forcing the flow throughout the system.

The arteries themselves are mere tubes. For instance, the hose to a sump pump is useless, that is without the pump. The arteries and heart have the same relationship. The difference is that the circulatory system has no outlet. This explains its vulnerability to high blood pressure: in other words, pressure in such a closed system can accumulate. When this occurs, it is an indication of underlying pathology, in other words, disease.

As long as the tube-like system, that is the arterial tree, is healthy the pressure remains normal. However, if the arteries become diseased—if they become blocked or narrowed—if they become inflamed, irritated, and scarred—then, the pressure will rise. Yet, despite the strain the pump must keep working. It must continue to move blood through the tightened or constricted arteries, which further weakens it. Ultimately, as a result of the strain it weakens, resulting in a heart attack.

It is critical to strengthen both the heart and arteries. This is the focus of the book. If this is achieved, hypertension will be cured.

If the arteries are healthy, the heart will also be healthy. Consider an automobile. It may be of the finest make with the most powerful engine, but it is useless, that is unless there are proper sturdy roads to travel on. Thus, it is critical to get the circulatory 'road map' in ideal health. This is achieved by first determining why the arteries are diseased. Then, those causes must be reversed. This is the only way to fully reverse this condition and, thus, ensure a long, vital, healthy life.

There are a number of factors which play a role in arterial disorders. Hormonal imbalances, vitamin deficiency, mineral deficiency, and various other factors are all critical. The role of such factors will be described. High blood pressure is a complicated disorder, and all related disorders must be evaluated as well as treated. Only then can this condition be permanently eradicated.

Traditionally, doctors regard diet as one of the most critical factors in high blood pressure, along with stress. Yet, physicians have no significant training in diet and nutrition. So, how could they understand the dietary connection?

For over fifty years the approach of the medical establishment has remained the same. The claim is the saturated fats found in animal foods, as well as cholesterol are the culprits. Salt is also blamed. The importance of stress is also implicated. Incredibly, none of these factors are the key players. The loss of flexibility—the arterial damage due to scarring and hardening—is the result of other culprits, which, usually, physicians fail to recognize.

With this condition the arteries are under siege. They are being attacked and poisoned. Cholesterol isn't the main attacker, nor is saturated fat, nor is salt. Such substances have formed a part of the human diet for untold thousands of years. Why wouldn't this disease have developed previously, that is in people who eat large amounts of cholesterol and/or saturates and even salt, for instance, the Bulgarians, Turks, the Azerbaijanis, Uzbeks, and Inuit? Hardening of the arteries and hypertension are modern diseases. There must be other factors, peculiar to the modern way of living, which are to blame.

Rees claims that patients must protect themselves from the development of stiff or hardened arteries. In this he is correct. Yet, he errs greatly in blaming dietary cholesterol and naturally occurring saturated fats, for instance, the fat of butter, whole milk, and red meat, as the cause. Then, he claims that restricting such foods from the diet will prevent the deposits, the so-called plaques or atheromas, which are associated with heart disease and high blood pressure. Thus, in order to prevent stiffening of the arteries he proposes that saturated fat and cholesterol must be restricted. Here, he makes a monumental error. The fact is cholesterol, as well as natural saturated fats, help keep the arterial walls elastic as well as smooth. Cholesterol is a wax that is needed for tissue repair. Such fats, in fact, prevent arterial degeneration.

Medical doctors receive no training in nutrition. In Dr. Rees's case this is evident. Actually, it is the refined and processed foods—the chemically contaminated foods, as well as beverages—which are destroying the arteries. These are the primary culprit. Such foods are the missing link explaining why primitive cultures and remote societies are free of these diseases, while in the Western world they are epidemic.

It is the sugar which destroys these organs, not the natural fats in, for instance, egg yolks, butter, cheese, milk, poultry, and red meat. Thus, regarding the diet for heart and high blood pressure patients there is good news. Eating the skin of chicken or turkey—even eating a large steak from a naturally raised cow—cannot cause stiffening of the arteries. The fact is such fatty foods are rich in the very nutrients these tissues need to stall this degeneration. In order to prevent such diseases there is a need to eat such rich foods. In contrast, soda pop, donuts, sweet rolls, pies, cakes, sugary cookies, candies, and deep fried foods cause arterial damage. Margarine stiffens the arteries, but butter doesn't. People are being misled—directly to the grave.

Few if any medical guides mention the main dietary culprit: refined sugar. If doctors emphasized the dangerous nature of this diabolical substance, this epidemic would be quickly reversed. What's more, food additives play a role in poisoning the circulatory system, as do refined and processed foods. Furthermore, the arteries, as well as the heart, are readily attacked by germs. The most significant of all factors may be the role played by infections in the cause of high blood pressure. (see Chapter 2).

There are also hormonal factors to consider, particularly dysfunction of the thyroid, pituitary, and adrenal glands. There are also nutritional deficiencies, that is the lack of vital components necessary for cellular functions—vitamins, minerals, essential fatty acids, and amino acids. Chronic toxicity is also a factor, for instance contamination by lead, cadmium, and solvents.

The toxicity of chlorine is a little mentioned factor. Even in the amount found in chlorinated water this substance aggressively damages the circulatory system, particularly the arteries. Yet, any volatile compound can cause arterial or heart damage.

Stress is also a major factor in such diseases. Severe stress causes the liberation of powerful compounds, particularly the steroid hormones. The liberation of excessive amounts of such hormones can result in a rise in blood pressure, arterial constriction, and even stroke or heart attack. Usually, there are other underlying factors. Yet, the fact is a sudden cardiovascular catastrophe can be precipitated by stress alone. For instance, consider the so-called white coat high blood pressure. This is where a person's blood pressure rises merely due to seeing their doctor. When such a person leaves the doctor's office, the blood pressure becomes lowered.

In developing a successful plan for the reversal of high blood pressure, as well as arterial disease, all these factors must be considered. Finally, the individual can be rid of this plague, simply by determining the causes and reversing them. That is the purpose of this book. It is not to cure this disease per se; it is to help guide the sufferer in the most productive direction possible. Yet, again, it is only a guide. The cure is up to you.

Chapter 1

Misconceptions Galore

Regarding the cause and cure for high blood pressure little has been written. This is despite the fact that this condition afflicts untold millions of people and causes uncountable millions of deaths yearly. In the medical profession no one seems to know what causes this disease. Yet, it is one of the primary causes of death in the Western world. Thus, the mystery remains unsolved.

Throughout the Western world heart and circulatory diseases account for a greater degree of death and disability than any other condition. It is about keeping this system in the most ideal health possible. It is also about how to reverse any existing disease. This is largely through arterial cleansing as well as the cleansing of toxins in general. It is through strengthening the function of the heart, while regenerating the structure of the arterial walls. It is also about purging all germs which cause inflammation.

It was Andrew Taylor Still, M.D., founder of the science of osteopathy, who first emphasized the importance of the arterial system, that network of arteries that reaches every region and organ in the body. He said that "The rule of the artery is supreme." In other words, all functions, and, thus, all aspects of health, are governed by the health of the arteries. Simply put, if the arteries are unhealthy, the entire body suffers. If they are healthy, the body is vitalized. Diseased arteries result in diseased tissues. Thus, it becomes obvious that for excellent health the arteries are the first place to begin.

The arteries are critical, because they control the most essential function of all: the delivery of nutrients and, particularly, oxygen, to the cells. Thus, they control the very essence of life. So, before any health plan can be instituted the arteries must be revitalized. This system must be thoroughly strengthened and cleansed. This will be achieved by following the plan in this book. It is a plan which relies exclusively on nature. This is because only nature provides the needed medicines and cures. Only a natural approach can heal. If the arteries are healthy, high blood pressure will fail to develop.

Drugs fail to heal the arteries. Rather, they poison them. There are no drugs which heal or cleanse the heart and arteries. There are no drugs which reverse heart disease. These substances only alter symptoms. Yet, the fact is there are numerous drugs, for instance, cortisone, aspirin, beta blockers, diuretics and alcohol, which damage the heart and/or arteries.

For Americans there is an apparent disregard for the needs of the body, including the circulatory system. With few exceptions people unwittingly assault their arteries through all manner of toxins: harsh drugs, alcohol, cigarette smoke, and refined foods, particularly white sugar, flour, and rice. It is the arterial system, along with the heart, which maintains vital health. If it degenerates, health dramatically declines.

People should seek to preserve and enhance these organs. They should take care of them. Rather than harming their organs in every conceivable way, they should nourish them. Every effort must be made to keep the heart and arteries in an ideal condition. It is the basis of existence: remember their rule is supreme.

Regarding arterial and heart disease, medicine takes a bizarre approach. Only the immediate problem is dealt with, for instance, a clot or narrowing in a specific artery or a weakness of a certain valve. In medicine the overall picture is neglected. No attempt is made to reverse the underlying cause. What's more, what sense is it to treat only a few inches of tissue—a mere few coronary arteries—when the entire system, thousands of miles long, is diseased? The fact is for ideal health the entire arterial tree must be cleansed: every inch of it. What's more, as a result there will be a total rejuvenation of the organ systems. The person will feel and look better than ever before. What's more, he/she will be rid of the burden of disease: permanently. That is the ultimate result of this program. The fact is through the careful adherence to the arterial cleaning system and heart-strengthening plan the vast majority of heart and arterial disorders will be eradicated, including high blood pressure.

Today, hypertension is perhaps the greatest of all epidemics. It is the only disease afflicting nearly one of three Americans. Incredibly, some 60 to 70 million North Americans suffer from this condition. What's more, medically, there is no hope for a cure. Among minorities hypertension is a major killer. In black males the incidence of this disease in certain areas may reach as high as 40%.

While it is a modern epidemic, this is far from a modern disease, with cases being recorded since antiquity. However, never before has it become an epidemic. Yet, as early as the 1950s physicians, such as Dr. Paul D. White, claimed this disease as the most important of all illnesses. This is because it is the most common of all illnesses which directly reduces life span.

This condition is known as the silent killer. This is because only rarely does it produce obvious symptoms. The fact is doctors frequently discover it only on a routine physical. An occasional mild headache or a sensation of fullness or tension in the head may be the only underlying symptoms.

Since the mid-1900s the incidence of inflammatory diseases of the arteries has also risen dramatically. Disorders, such as vasculitis, arteritis, and phlebitis, that is internal blood clots, are virtually epidemic. High blood pressure is particularly important, because of the vast number of diseases associated with it. All such diseases are potentially fatal. All ultimately result in diseased arteries as well as a weakened or diseased heart.

High blood pressure is a major cause of enlarged heart syndrome. If prolonged and untreated, it also leads to kidney damage. In some individuals uncontrolled high blood pressure causes lung damage, a condition known as pulmonary hypertension. Obviously, unchecked hypertension is often a catastrophe, since it damages the body's most critical organs. The brain may also be negatively affected, particularly its blood vessels. Here, inflammation and obstructions may develop, as well as scarring, leading to stroke. What's more, the arterial walls may become weakened, which can lead to aneurysms. This may result in bleeding within the brain, which is usually fatal.

Most people are unaware of the causes of high blood pressure. Even most doctors are clueless. In most instances people simply take the prescribed medication, without even considering the true cause. Yet, the medications never address the cause. Incredibly, the vast majority of people with this illness are classified into a bizarre category. This category is called "essential" hypertension. This simply means that the cause is unknown. No attempt is made to determine it, the approach being merely to prescribe medication to forcibly reduce the blood pressure.

In a smaller percentage, perhaps 5% to 10%, the cause may be determined. Here, the pathology or symptoms are so obvious that the physician is able to make a diagnosis of a specific disease, for instance, the hypertension of Cushing's Syndrome , kidney tumors, scarred lungs (pulmonary hypertension), adrenal tumors (pheochromocytoma), and similar rare or remote disorders. These are the exceptions. The vast majority never get an adequate diagnosis.

The purpose of this book is to describe the true causes of hypertension, in all its types, while recommending the proper therapy. The therapy is strictly natural: no drugs. This is because it is diet, herbal therapy, and various natural substances, which reverse this disorder. Again, hypertension can be reversed, even the more pathological types. The key is to apply an approach which reverses the underlying cause, which is usually acute or chronic infection. Another major cause is nutritional deficiency. Yet, even with the latter there is usually an associated hidden infection.

In general the medical profession refuses to admit that its approach is faulty. Yet, in hypertension the approach is not only faulty, but it is also dangerous. This reminds me of the time when I was an intern, and saw a horrible catastrophe. The presiding doctor, a general practitioner, was always jealous of me. I tried to keep a low profile, because the doctors wanted me harmed. I had already been threatened for helping a patient avoid drugs and surgery and for curing her with vitamin therapy. So, pathetically, I was forced to watch the devilish deed unfold: a woman, who was highly emotional and quite thin, was subject to bouts of high blood pressure. When these bouts occurred, her husband would often bring her to the hospital.

They were a tense couple: I knew that all that was necessary was relaxation, along with aggressive nutritional therapy, for instance, intravenous magnesium and B vitamins. The general practitioner, in his self-righteousness, insisted on forcing the blood pressure down. Intravenously, he gave a high dose of a potent and rather new anti-hypertensive drug. Instinctively, I became concerned, realizing the potential consequences of forcibly lowering blood pressure. Unfortunately, my instincts were correct. To my horror the blood pressure dropped too quickly; there was no way the body could adjust. As a result, she suffered a stroke, strictly due to the drug. Now she was relegated to a wheel chair, her husband pushing her to and fro in the hospital. He cried out one day, "Now look at my wife—look at what you left me with." This was the legacy of those dire days during my hospital rotation: one vile catastrophe after another, which could have been largely prevented had a more natural, in fact, cause-and-effect, approach been taken.

Here is what I would have done in this case. I would have talked to the couple gently and given them reassurance. Then, I would have ordered a gentle massage of the spine and feet with calming essential oils, while also prescribing natural medicines which calm the nervous system, particularly royal jelly and rosemary. I would have given her large amounts of unprocessed red sour grape (Resvital) sublingually, along with the special herbal formula for high blood pressure, Hyper-10. As a special means to ease her toxicity I would have given her Royal Oil under the tongue. This women appeared to be septic. So, also, I would have given her a potent natural germicide such as the OregaBiotic. I would have also checked the health of her gums to see if there were pockets of infection. Then, I would have dispensed the special multiple spice gum treatment, the OregaDENT. All this would have naturally lowered blood pressure, while strengthening the blood vessel walls. Thus, a human catastrophe would have been prevented. Regarding the diet the intake of sweets would have been prohibited. Intravenously, magnesium, pantothenic acid, and vitamin C would have been administered. Thus, this stroke could have been prevented.

This is why I am writing this book: to avoid further catastrophes. It is because of the fact that there are answers: there are ways to prevent human agony. Rather than in drug therapy answers are found in nature. Nature, that is the powers of God almighty, provides an enormous number of substances, which help reverse heart and/or arterial disease. Many such substances act directly upon the heart. For instance, consider the most often-used heart drug: digitalis. It is exclusively a natural compound, derived from a kind of weed: the foxglove. Incredibly, the flower of the foxglove is a brilliant blood-red. This can be no coincidence—it is a sign that this plant is good for the heart. It is evidence of a higher power, which creates the code for existence, the very substances which humans, as well as animals, require. How else would the precise medicine humans need be automatically available? In other words, these substances pre-exist for human, as well as animal, needs.

Humans didn't make these natural medicines. Yet, they work perfectly within the human body. There could only be one source for such a system, and it is far from mere blind chaos, mere uncontrolled evolution. There must be a Master Mind, who developed all for human benefit. Call this Mind what you will, from a scientific point of view there is little doubt that such a Being exists. The fact is evidence exists that these very medicines were created specifically for human use, because they act directly upon the various organ systems, improving their function. Natural medicines cure high blood pressure.

Synthetic ones fail to do so. Natural medicines heal the tissues, without serious side effects. Synthetic drugs may alter symptoms, but they do so while causing tissue damage.

In modern medicine there is a kind of apathy. The fact is there is utter pessimism. Regarding disease doctors rarely take a positive attitude. Consumed by indifference the average physician is static, failing to take any action to combat and/or reverse disease. Only a minority of physicians pursue the true causes of disease. Even a lesser number search for cures. This is largely because of the philosophy of modern medicine, that is to "treat the symptoms" rather than the cause. Yet, incredibly, in ancient times there was a voluminous attempt to discern the cause, largely because physicians were interested in discovering cures.

The medical system is hopelessly inadequate in reversing common diseases. Yet, natural medicines are highly capable of doing so. In contrast, consider the medical approach for any disease, for instance, heart disease, arterial disorders, congestive heart failure, and high blood pressure. Are cures ever offered? Are patients ever told that if they take a specific approach, that is with diet and herbal medicine, along with, perhaps, exercise, their diseases will be eradicated? By the average physician are they ever given instructions on how they may reduce or halt their medication(s)? No such approaches are provided. The fact is regarding chronic or degenerative diseases modern medicine fails to offer even a single cure.

In the Western world high blood pressure causes uncountable deaths. Stroke, which is secondary to it, yearly kills tens of thousands of Americans. Hypertension-induced kidney disease kills thousands of Americans yearly. What's more, diabetics frequently die from high blood pressure-related complications. Yet, for all such diseases no cures are provided. Nor are any preventive measures advised. This book gives the precise cures, plus prevention.

There is the right diet for fighting these diseases. Plus, the substances which must be avoided are clarified. What's more, the exact natural medicines needed to eliminate these plagues are described. Even the precise dosages are given. Plus, the ideal brand names are listed. All that is necessary is described.

One reason there has been little if any progress in this disease relates to the government. Here, the so-called authorities, who are usually lobbyists, have a one-track mind. They continue to emphasize outdated or infective approaches such as salt restriction and medication. This is despite the fact that such an approach is obviously faulty; the incidence of hypertension is dramatically rising. What's more, recent data shows that salt restriction offers no benefit in reversing or even preventing this disease. The severe salt restriction practiced by innumerable individuals diagnosed with hypertension, the incredibly bland diet, which they so assiduously follow, is all for naught. Critical factors, such as the role of chronic infection, gum disease, nutritional deficiency, inflammatory diseases, dietary faddism, and hormonal disorders, are rarely if ever discussed.

Despite evidence to the contrary the government maintains its position: for individuals diagnosed with hypertension a salt restricted diet is mandatory. Since when did the government become licensed to practice medicine? The fact is it is the government, which purposely provides disinformation despite the latest research, which proves otherwise.

There is now clear evidence that severe salt restriction fails to reverse this disease and in some instances aggravates it. Yet, the government blindly maintains this theory, that is that dietary salt and saturated fat are the culprits. What's more, regarding natural cures little if any information is provided, even though the curative properties of such substances are well established. Thus, people must search for the cures on their own.

The wisdom of civilizations

In the late 1990s during international travels I made a first-ever observation. People who live vital and long lives had one thing in common. They regularly consume antiseptic herbs or foods in the diet. What's more, people who are free from heart disease, as well as high blood pressure, have another common habit: they regularly consume flavonoid-rich fruit, particularly grapes. In other words, as a result of their native diets they are unwittingly warding off disease.

I began to wonder: why would hot spices prevent the major killers of modern time: heart disease, high blood pressure, diabetes, and cancer? Why are the people, who regularly consume antiseptic spices, relatively free of this disease?

In a sense it might be thought that such spices would agitate the nerves, raising blood pressure. Yet, people who regularly consume them have the lowest incidence of high blood pressure in the world. For instance, in India, Sri Lanka, Malaysia, Turkey, and Greece, especially the primitive areas, high blood pressure is rare. There must be a connection which was never previously considered.

Why are the primitives, who take natural grape tonics and/or eat mountain-grown grapes, as well as other Mediterranean fruit, such as pomegranates, relatively free of this deadly plague? Why are Americans so afflicted, who eat mainly other types of fruit, such as apples, commercial berries, pears, commercial grapes, tomatoes, pineapple, bananas, etc.? Obviously, for Americans these are missing factors. For people in the West it is necessary to uncover these factors. It is crucial to include such protective substances in the daily regimen. Only then can high blood pressure and all its consequences thoroughly be cured.

Yet, what of these villagers, who rarely if ever suffer from this plague? In my investigations in these villages the only ones who had the disease were heavy drinkers, and even their hypertension was relatively mild. Yet, the villagers who were protecting themselves didn't do so intentionally.

It is just their way. They fail to consider that their habits will make them live longer or free them of disease. Yet, the fact is it is possible to learn from them and reap the benefits.

Regarding germ-killing foods, as well as spices, in many foreign lands the consumption is vast. This is important, because, as this book will elucidate, germs play a major role in hypertension. These villagers are largely in the Mediterranean and Middle East: Bulgaria, Turkey, Syria, Greece, Iraq, Iran, Pakistan, India, and Lebanon. They consume germ-killing foods or beverages, because they like the taste. Raw unfiltered honey, raw vinegar, garlic, onions, shallots, leeks, sage, cilantro, radishes, turnips, hot-tasting greens, hot peppers, cumin, hot sauces and pastes, curry powder, mint, and oregano are consumed plentifully and regularly. I noticed one villager commonly had a routine of eating spicy hot greens in large quantities with virtually every meal. He claimed he never was sick. Others routinely drank sage and oregano tea.

Yogurt, with its vast germ-fighting capacities, is regularly consumed. Fresh yogurt is made from raw or even boiled milk free of hormones or GMO material. It is on the daily menu of most villagers. In the cities it is either fresh or pasteurized. In both cases it is loaded with healthy cultures, giving the intestines vital and disease-preventing quantities of healthy bacteria. What's more, evidence exists that the natural bacteria help prevent high blood pressure. Plus, yogurt is a rich source of calcium. The calcium in yogurt is readily absorbed, and this mineral combats high blood pressure.

Black tea, a mild antiseptic, up to 10 cups daily, is a staple. Although, it is corrupted by the addition of prodigious amounts of sugar. Then, there are the glorious herbal teas, not the weak, devitalized commercially available types common in the West, which have lost their aromatic essences. Instead, the actual sprigs fresh from the mountains or the freshly ground herb are used. Such mountain-fresh teas are rich in potent aromatic compounds. It is the aromatic substances which provide germicidal actions and which are responsible for the low incidence of high blood pressure. Without them the teas are ineffective as immune or circulatory tonics. The fresh aroma and taste of aromatic compounds are common in the untarnished village teas; how completely novel from the Western experience it is. It is a daily routine; hardly anyone misses a dose. Essentially, if you are a guest it is "forced" upon you.

There are also the hot and spicy foods, so hot that many Westerners could never eat them. These foods, spiced with hot peppers, curry powder, cumin, oregano, cinnamon, cloves, and more, help block the development of heart disease and high blood pressure.

The American diet is notoriously bland. Many Americans avoid eating spicy fair. They claim they cannot tolerate it, that it upsets their digestion, and that their systems are too sensitive to consume it. They may even claim that spices damage their stomachs, perhaps causing actual illnesses, like heartburn and ulcers. Yet, there is no evidence that spicy foods cause such disorders. Rather, it is the bland foods, such as white bread, white rice, and white sugar, which are responsible.

Spices dramatically stimulate immunity. What's more, they greatly stimulate the production of digestive juices, which is necessary for normal digestion. Such juices help prevent disconcerting digestive symptoms such as bloating, spasticity, heartburn, and diarrhea. In contrast, bland foods create these symptoms, increasing the risks for the development of gastritis, esophagitis, and ulcers. Yet, for the majority of Americans spicy foods are vigorously shunned. As a result, the non-spice eaters are highly vulnerable to a variety of diseases, since spices are among the richest sources of potent biological substances known, which protect the body from disease. Bland foods stall digestion. Spicy foods encourage it.

Again, consider the American diet, so rich in relatively bland foods such as white sugar, candies, cookies, cakes, pies, donuts, sweet rolls, bagels, bread, rolls, buns, crackers, cheese, well done meat, milk, potatoes, overdone vegetables, and cereal. Such a diet is directly responsible for the development of digestive disturbances, including gastric ulcer, duodenal ulcer, Crohn's disease, spastic colon, constipation, diverticulitis, and ulcerative colitis. It is also responsible for the degeneration of the heart and arteries, which leads to high blood pressure.

It is easy to understand why Americans are vulnerable. With the exception of ethnic populations, who consume their traditional foods, it is rarely spicy. None of the typical American foods offer even the slightest degree of antiseptic power, with the exception of perhaps Mexican- or Italian-style fare. Rather, such foods encourage the growth of microbes.

A teaspoon of white sugar is sufficient to halt the function of billions of white blood cells, while causing the growth of billions of yeasts. Imagine what happens if a person consumes it by the tablespoonful daily. The fact is there are some Americans who consume as much as a cup of sugar daily as hidden or obvious calories. For instance, a single soda has some seven teaspoonfuls of this deadly substance. A donut has up to ten teaspoons. Two donuts plus coffee with sugar causes absolute sugar overload, a meal guaranteed to cause harm.

Anyone who consumes large quantities of this poison is simultaneously feeding germs, which cause chronic immune suppression, as well as infections, especially by yeasts. The fact is the consumption of the equivalent of a single tablespoonful (three teaspoons) of refined sugar is sufficient to generate the growth of tens of billions of yeasts and molds within the body. This explains the significant immunosuppressive actions of this substance. The fact is the body regards refined sugar as a poison. Thus, its consumption should be strictly avoided.

Kids are major sugar eaters. This extensive sugar ingestion greatly weakens their immune systems, making them vulnerable to microbial attack. Due to their faulty diets, many children are microbial breweries, overpopulated by untold trillions of disease-causing germs. Thus, they become a sort of living microbial incubator, seeding infections to any near them. If a pandemic strikes, such individuals will be exceptionally vulnerable. So will those who care for them. Thus, their diets must be radically improved. Otherwise, they may well die in vast numbers. The fact is refined sugar is a major cause of a wide range of cardiovascular diseases, including hypertension. In children a history of major sugar consumption is directly tied to the development of hypertension as an adult.

Clearly, the high sugar intake increases the risk for the development of diabetes and adult-onset diseases, particularly cardiovascular disorders. Professor John Yudkin of London's Queen's Hospital in London, England clearly proved that high sugar intake is the major cause of heart and arterial diseases. He described an ominous finding among dead soldiers during the Korean War. Upon autopsy these 20-or-so-year-old men were found to have the arteries of 50 to 60-year-olds, which was directly attributed to their high sugar intake.

Heart disease: an infection?

Regarding all forms of heart disease from the medical point of view emphasis is on diet. Here, the effort has been to reduce salt and fat intake. Cholesterol and saturated fats are deemed the culprits. No one ever considered any other cause. Medical textbooks strictly emphasize the role of salt and, thus, the need for dietary restriction. There is rarely if ever any mention of an infectious cause. There is the occasional mention of sudden or toxic infection as a factor, particularly in high blood pressure. However, for medical professionals the fact that this condition is caused by various chronic infections, not diet, is virtually unthinkable. Yet, the medical literature is replete with supporting evidence. There are a plethora of scientific studies, which document an infectious role. Germs which commonly infect the heart and arteries include herpes, chlamydia, staph, strep, nanobacteria, and candida.

The miracle of blood

Every day the circulatory system performs perhaps the greatest miracle of all: it delivers blood to all organs, keeping them alive and functioning. It is crucial to know just what blood is. It is the medium of life; it is an organ in its own right. In fact, it is a fluid, active, moving organ. Consider this: no organ in the body can survive without it. Thus, it is of equal importance as the heart, liver, or brain. The fact is these organs depend upon the blood for their survival.

Blood is the essence of existence. It is well known that when an excess of blood is lost, a person can develop severe brain damage. Death may even result. Bound by the arteries it is a closed system. Thus, it is an internal organ. This fact is important in understanding the nature of hypertension. Because of its closed nature any toxic insult can readily destabilize it, potentially leading to inflammation, infection, tissue damage, and, ultimately, high blood pressure. High blood pressure is the end-stage manifestation of such damage and toxicity. Since it is a closed circuit, toxins can't easily be removed. Thus, such toxins may readily cause the damage which results in blood pressure elevation.

The majority of these toxins are microbial in nature, although synthetic poisons, including heavy metals, also play a major role. Yet, other organs, which regulate blood pressure, may also be poisoned. These organs include the pituitary, thyroid, and adrenal glands. For the blood pressure to return to normal the function of these organs must also be restored. In some instances disorders of the glandular system are the primary cause of high blood pressure. This further demonstrates the importance of detoxification.

The blood is a living tissue and the only one which is exclusively fluid. This fluid must be kept in optimal health in order to avoid disease. What's more, in the reversal of hypertension the health of blood must be considered. Here, any infections must be destroyed. Plus, the blood must be purged of toxins. Both of these approaches must be administered simultaneously for optimal results to be achieved.

As is confirmed by uncountable medical texts the heart is easily infected by germs, as are the arteries. Thus, it is likely that the cause of a specific case of heart or arterial trouble is infective. This means that for many people diagnosed with arterial narrowing, including coronary artery disease, the wrong approach has been taken. The first approach is to eradicate any infections. Surgery is the most extreme option, in fact, the last resort. First, hidden infections must be cleansed. What's more, accumulations of toxins, including solvents and heavy metals, must be purged.

Surgery spreads infections. It worsens toxicity. Thus, again, this is only the most extreme and last resort and should never be undergone merely for "prevention." Certainly, for high blood pressure the surgical options are limited.

Blood cleansing: ancient technique, modern value

Today, no one considers the importance of clean, healthy blood. People often attempt to cleanse their colons and livers. However, in general the health of the bloodstream is neglected. In the early 1900s this was not the case. Then, entire clinics specialized in blood cleansing. Products and tonics, specifically for cleansing the blood, were produced and marketed. People realized the dangers of unhealthy blood and the benefits of purifying it. The importance of blood cleansing can be demonstrated by a simple fact. Within minutes whatever enters it travels to every cell and organ in the body. Thus, the health of human cells and organs are directly dependent upon the health of the blood. If the blood is diseased, all cells will be affected. If it is healthy, all cells and organs will correspond. If it is septic, the entire body will become septic, even critical organs such as the brain, kidneys, liver, and heart. What's more, if it is toxic, so will be the rest of the body.

Everyone knows that blood is red. This is because of the interaction of oxygen with the iron-containing protein known as hemoglobin. The oxygen is derived from the air which flows through the lungs. The hemoglobin is produced in the bone marrow, spleen, and liver. Untold trillions of red cells are found in the body, and each is responsible for transporting oxygen to the cells. Thus, the red cells are critical to human survival. Without them death rapidly ensues. These cells must be kept in the most optimal health possible. To do so toxins must be cleansed from the body as well as invasive germs.

Blood-letting is a simple technique to achieve this. Blood holds the toxins. By simply removing a quantity of blood the levels of toxins are significantly reduced. This may result in a revitalization of health. If indicated, see your doctor about possible blood-letting. This remedy was popularized by the Prophet Muhammad and is highly effective for cardiovascular disorders. He recommended this primarily as a preventive medicine.

Oxygen: nature's germ killer

The brightness of the blood is an indication of its health. It is a sign of a high level of oxygenation. Purplish blood is normal, but only in the veins. If the arterial blood is dark or purplish, it may be a sign of low oxygen. This is typical in lung diseases, where the oxygen-delivering capacity of the lungs is compromised.

As long as the lungs can absorb oxygen from the air, the health of the body will remain intact. The red cells, with the miraculous pigment known as hemoglobin, will readily absorb the oxygen and deliver it to the tissues. However, if the lungs are unable to provide sufficient oxygen, the health of the tissues will suffer. For instance, the arteries and heart may fail to get sufficient oxygen, and, thus, they become weakened. This may lead to chronic infection. What's more, germs thrive in a low oxygen environment, while, in contrast, their growth is inhibited by high or normal levels.

In a low oxygen environment there is a strain upon the heart and arteries; the heart is forced to work excessively, which places great strain upon it. What's more, when the oxygen content is low, the arteries begin to degenerate. Thus, in the development of high blood pressure lung disease may play a role.

Yet, there is another way the process can be disturbed: toxic gases, in particular, carbon monoxide. The latter is particularly dangerous, because on a cellular level it mimics oxygen. The red blood cells are unable to discriminate between it and oxygen. Thus, if the body is exposed to this gas, the red cells quickly go into action. They bind the gas, reducing but never eliminating its toxicity. The fact is this binding is highly dangerous. In effect, carbon monoxide causes oxygen starvation. If there is significant exposure, the many trillions of red blood cells can be poisoned; they cannot quickly release this aggressive gas to regain oxygen. Thus, the tissues become oxygen starved.

The brain has a high need for oxygen; the carbon monoxide poisoning shuts off oxygen flow to the brain, resulting in drowsiness, then unconsciousness. If there is no ventilation and the if gas levels build up, severe oxygen starvation may result, leading to death. Every year this happens to hundreds of Americans. Yet, there is another debacle: chronic carbon monoxide poisoning. This may result from leaky appliances, poor ventilation, or job-related exposure. The chronic toxicity ultimately damages the circulatory system, leading to high blood pressure.

For the blood pressure disorder to be cured the source of the gas must be ascertained and the exposure eliminated. The blood and organs must be cleansed of toxins and the health of the red cells revived. This can be achieved through a healthy diet rich in organic greens, which are oxygenating. Certain supplements help cleanse the blood, while increasing oxygenation. Such supplements include the GreensFlush wild greens extract, oil of wild oregano, Resvital crude red grape powder, and juice of wild oregano. All these are effective in halting carbon monoxide toxicity. Natural vitamin C also helps neutralize the toxicity. The natural type is the kind found in Purely-C.

The medical profession claims such poisoning is incurable. With potent natural medicines, such as the wild greens, the oregano juice, and the Resvital, virtually any case of carbon monoxide poisoning can be reversed, that is if the supplementation is given soon enough and repeatedly.

Toxic blood means a toxic heart and arteries: how to cleanse the blood

Throughout this book information will be provided regarding blood cleansing. If the blood is sick, so will be the heart and arteries. This has to be so. These organs, like all others, are dependent upon it. If the blood is clean, that is if it is purged of all toxic irritants, there could be no hypertension. The wild greens, crude red grape, wild oregano juice, and various wild oregano-based germ killers are the ideal agents for purging the blood of toxins as well as germs.

To complete the cleansing a kind of roto-rooter-like action is required. This is to cleanse any thickenings, inflammations, and clots. It is also to aggressively cleanse the arterial lining of any hardenings, i.e. atheromas. This is accomplished through the intake of potent natural enzymes, which are specific for decontaminating the arteries. For such enzymes Infla-eez is ideal. This contains the highest grade fruit-source enzymes, with great digestive/cleansing capacities.

Infla-eez is the ideal natural "roto-rooter" for the arteries. This is because it is contains only fruit-source enzymes, which are fully edible and which can be taken in large quantities. Plus, the enzymes in this formula have proven biological activity. This is a special blend of unprocessed raw enzymes from the stems of pineapples, green papayas, and green papaya seeds. The seed extract, which is organic, is highly biologically active and is only available in a limited supply. All the enzymes in Infla-eez are highly biologically active. Thus, a roto-rooter action is assured. Infla-eez is invaluable for reversal of lymphatic blockages, for instance, cellulite, swellings in the legs, and lymphedema. This supplement works best when taken with water on an empty stomach.

Inflammation is now regarded as a prime cause of heart and arterial disease. In high blood pressure there is systemic inflammation. Infla-eez helps purge this. If taken regularly along with other key nutritional supplements, it will help prevent inflammatory reactions within the tissues. Note: this is similar to another formula known as Infla-eez. However, Infla-eez is specially formulated to purge obstructions from the arteries.

Today, drugs are correlated with an increase in inflammation, even an increase in the incidence. Consider this: for inflammation Infla-eez can be taken without the risks for side effects. There is no possibility that this substance can cause, for instance, blood clots, strokes, and heart attacks.

With fruit-based enzymes there are no side effects. In fact, these enzymes offer powers which are useful in reversing obstructions, including blood clots. The fact is the regular intake of such substances results in an improvement of overall health. Since it is fully natural and, in fact, is a food, the Infla-eez can be taken over a prolonged period, that is however long it takes to resolve the problem. This is equally as effective as coumadin only it is natural— without any negative effects. See your doctor about using natural foods as blood thinners instead of dangerous drugs. Do not take both together. Only one approach should be selected: either the drugs or the natural foods such as Infla-eez, Resvital, wild oregano, and Purely-C.

High blood pressure: a sign of a weak heart?

People are of the belief that high blood pressure means the heart is pumping hard. In many instances, this is certainly true, but what is little understood is that, overall, the heart is weakened. This largely explains the development of high blood pressure: the arteries are compensating for a weak heart. Thus, in order for high blood pressure to be cured the heart must be strengthened. Only through such an approach can the high blood pressure be fully reversed. This is because, again, this disorder is a compensation for a weak heart. When the heart loses strength, the arteries compensate, that is they become taut. Thus, the circulatory system is a single unit. In order to reverse disease all components of this unit must be treated. A strong heart means a normal blood pressure.

Infection can weaken the heart. Virtually any germ can infect this organ. One relatively unknown factor is parasites. In heart disease the likelihood for parasitic infection of the heart is relatively high. This is particularly true for individuals with weak and enlarged hearts. The enlargement may be a signal of infestation by parasites, which attack the heart muscle. One such parasite is, incredibly, the dog heartworm. There are potentially millions of Americans whose hearts are infected by this parasite. Close contact with a dog is usually the source. However, blood transfusions may also play a role.

For the heart to regain its strength and, therefore, for the blood pressure to be normalized, the infection(s) must be eradicated. This can be achieved through the use of potent herbs, spices, and foods, which strengthen heart muscle function and which also destroy any invasive germs. Here, the primary cures are the edible oil of wild oregano (P73) and the OregaBiotic. The OregaBiotic is a special form of wild spice extracts combining four unique spice oils. It is capable of killing the entire gamut of germs, which cause cardiovascular disease. This will regenerate the heart's strength. Yet, this organ will also be strengthened by reviving the glands, a subject covered in Chapter 5.

Why high blood pressure (hypertension) is important

With high blood pressure there is an increased risk for a wide range of diseases. Even mild high blood pressure usually lowers life expectancy, that is if it remains uncorrected. Correction via drugs usually fails to improve life expectancy. In fact, such drugs are a major cause of sudden death, that is they increase the death rate.

Even so, untreated severe hypertension is a crisis. It is a catastrophe, which is looming. When the blood pressure is volatile, there is a high risk for serious disease as well as sudden death. In particular, according to the AMA's *Family Medical Guide* untreated so-called malignant high blood pressure, that is the type that is persistently high and out of control, may result in sudden death within six months. Yet, if the patient adheres to preventive advice through a natural approach, all could be corrected. This is true even of the most dire cases.

Even so, it is understandable that doctors feel the need to react. They know that if they fail to do so and the patient develops a complication, for instance, a massive stroke, they are liable. What's more, many are sincere in their attempts to "save the patient" through rather extreme measures. Yet, the entire approach is misguided. The fact is the patient is rarely if ever saved. At best, all that is treated are the symptoms. The underlying disease and, therefore, the danger, remain. No cures are achieved.

What is definitely known is that as a result of high blood pressure, the heart works harder. The heart is a pump. Like any pump, eventually, it wears out. The greater the amount of friction it must pump against—and hypertension is the result of excess friction—the sooner it will give out. In other words, the heart must work against this resistance, which ultimately causes it to thicken or enlarge, much as a machine part will become damaged as a result of excess work. The pressure can be so great that the heart may gradually or even suddenly fail. Thus, the friction must be reduced, so that the heart can remain viable as long as possible. This demonstrates why it is crucial to eradicate this disease and do so quickly. There is no time to waste. The fact is in North America alone some 100,000 people die yearly as a consequence of this disease.

Yet, it is the gradual degeneration of the arteries, which is of such great concern. Then, as a consequence the heart degenerates. Hypertension is merely the end-stage of this degeneration. The arteries begin to decay first, which leads to this disease. Decay or degeneration of the arteries is a sign of aging. At all costs the arteries must be kept healthy.

Healthy arteries facilitate a rapid cure for any disease. This system is known medically as the arterial tree. It is the system used by the body to deliver the nutrients, as well as medicines, required by all cells. These structures, that is this entire arterial tree, must be cleansed. Any inflammation, as well as infection, must be reversed. It makes no sense to attempt to cure or treat only a tiny segment of this tree, such as a few coronary arteries. For health to be restored the entire system must be purged as well as regenerated.

Hypertension is the result of diseased arteries. It is a warning sign, as if to say, "The insides of your arteries are diseased and must be cleansed." High blood pressure is a warning of the true condition of these structures, that is the fact that they are decaying, inflamed, probably infected, and hardened. Ultimately, this will affect all organs, as all of these structures are supplied by arteries. What's more, certain organs, notably the brain and kidneys, contain a vast network of arteries, and these are among the main organs damaged as a result of this disease.

Again, what must be remembered is that this disease isn't merely the obvious, that is "elevated blood pressure." It is a warning of systemic disease. That is it tells of the existence of total circulatory disease, not just of the heart and main arteries but of all arteries throughout the body—thousands of miles of them. It also warns of disease of the internal organs. The heart, arteries, kidneys, and brain are mainly involved but all other organs are also negatively affected.

Pomerantz in his book, *Family Physician,* provides a reminder of the seriousness of this disease. As a result of high blood pressure he claims that to a degree all tissues suffer damage and changes. This implies that high blood pressure causes systemic damage. Every day this condition persists there will be a greater degree of cellular damage and death. No organ is immune. Thus, every effort must be made not only to merely to control the blood pressure but also to fully normalize it. This is done by eradicating the true cause of the condition, and the methods for this will be described throughout this book. The point is the body is supposed to have a normal blood pressure: for life. Any elevation above the norm is a warning of internal damage. The damage can only get worse over time. Unless the process is halted the only consequence is fulminant disease as well as premature death.

Chapter 2

The Infection Connection

There is seemingly an infectious nature in virtually all diseases. For instance, consider chronic stomach disorders, including ulcers. These have been proven to be caused largely by a bacterial infection, the notorious *Helicobacter pylori*. Also, consider multiple sclerosis, which was once regarded as cause unknown. Now it is known that the nerve sheaths of multiple sclerosis sufferers are infected by herpes viruses. The viruses apparently destroy the nerve sheath, leading to this syndrome. Another example is cancer. It has clearly been shown that a high percentage of cancerous tumors are infected with viruses and/or parasites, even molds and yeasts. Thus, regardless of the disease there appears to be an infectious agent. The same is true of high blood pressure. This is because germs have been found in people with this condition. What's more, such germs are in general not found in people with normal blood pressure.

It is well known that high blood pressure is directly associated with kidney disease, particularly kidney infections. This disease has also been directly tied to dental infections, as will be demonstrated in this chapter. Furthermore, the fact that high blood pressure patients suffer from inflammatory diseases is also well known. Inflammation is usually caused by infection. The infectious agent can be bacterial, fungal, viral, or parasitic.

That infection could be a major factor should be no surprise, especially when studying the severe nature of the arterial damage. Obviously, in this condition the arteries are under great stress, and they are extensively damaged. Surely, such arteries are under attack. Germs are the likely culprits.

Arterial wall damage: a proven fact

In high blood pressure it is well established that the arterial walls are damaged. For decades surgeons have observed bizarre damage on the inside of the arteries. The arteries are stiff; their normal elasticity is lost. Scar formation occurs, and the scarred and/or damaged areas are often infiltrated with cholesterol as well as calcium.

The existence of cholesterol deposits within the arterial walls has been a source of great confusion. It has led many to believe that, incredibly, cholesterol is the cause of heart/arterial disease. The fact is this view was the source for the now-in-vogue low cholesterol diets. True, there is cholesterol within the arteries. It is a major component of plaque. However, consider this: cholesterol is a wax, that is a sealant. The body uses it to seal, that is wall off, damage. It is the ideal agent for sealing arterial damage to prevent bleeding. Thus, cholesterol is far from the cause of this disease, in fact, it is part of the cure.

High cholesterol diets have never been proven to cause high blood pressure. Diets high in pork and/or nitrated meats are certainly associated, but this is not because of the cholesterol content. It is more greatly related to the fact that pork contains a wide range of parasites and germs, which can invade the heart and arteries, causing inflammation. In other words, microbially, it is filthy. What's more, nitrates cause a violent kind of poisoning, which can lead to a wide range of degenerative diseases, including high blood pressure, angina, heart attack, heart failure, arthritis, rheumatoid arthritis, viral infections, and cancer. Nitrates also destroy vitamin C, which is needed to prevent arterial wall damage. Thus, by oxidizing vitamin C, the key substance involved in the formation of the arteries' elastic membranes, nitrates cause extensive damage. With a severe or prolonged lack of this vitamin, combined with the regular intake of nitrates, the arterial walls stiffen and become scarred.

The arterial system is vast. Thus, large amounts of vitamin C are needed on a regular basis to keep it in ideal health. The vitamin C is needed for repair, a constant issue with arteries, which are routinely subject to damage. Only the naturally occurring type can be relied upon for tissue healing, that is the type found in food and food extracts. For nutritional supplements and food concentrates, which are rich in naturally occurring vitamin C, see Appendix A. Note: a reasonable dosage for protection is 200 to 300 mg daily of natural vitamin C.

In my early training I remember well the bizarre damage that was observable within human arteries—the result of toxic ways of living. Every North American has diseased arteries. During surgery it was common to find a kind of necrotic residue, which was malodorous, on the inside of the arteries. This residue is a sign of severe toxicity, in fact, infection. As mentioned previously hypertension is merely the final manifestation of such damage. This is because the damage develops over a period of decades, all largely due to the consumption of processed foods, particularly refined sugar, nitrated meats, and toxic fats. Pork products are also directly related.

I attended several cardiovascular surgeries to gain an understanding of the pathology. In one case, an operation known as a carotid endarterectomy, where the carotid arteries are "cleaned out" and replaced with artificial structures, the evidence was clear. When conducting this surgery, the huge arteries in the neck, the carotid arteries, were opened. The diseased arteries were removed and replaced with artificial types. In the patient the arteries were filled with necrotic residue, which was obviously the result of extreme inflammation. The inner linings of the arteries were scarred. A kind of septic-appearing residue was scraped out. The fact is it was clearly infective in nature. The scarring within the arteries also appeared to have an infective cause.

The surgeons were not interested in such a theory. They never even made mention of this obvious finding. Now it is clear that infection plays a significant role and that, in fact, it may be the primary factor. The fact is a wide range of germs have been found to actively infect the arteries. What's more, these are chronic infections, not the types which can be successfully treated with antibiotics, but, rather, must be cured through a more comprehensive approach.

Typically, with aging the major arteries of the body undergo a degree of scarring. This is especially true in individuals diagnosed with atherosclerosis, that is hardening of the arteries. Infection is the likely explanation for the scar formation seen in people with this condition. The fact that a person's arteries are scarified with aging is an ominous finding. This process must be stopped, that is if good health is expected.

Yet, the greatest factor of all, which damages the arteries, is sugar. A no-sugar diet helps keep the arteries healthy. On such a diet these organs rarely degenerate, and, as a result, life expectancy is increased. In contrast, the regular intake of refined sugar leads to a vast degree of cardiovascular damage and, therefore, a reduction in life expectancy. The arteries are greatly damaged, as is the heart muscle itself. This damage is caused by a phenomenon known as cross-linking. Here, the sugar molecules attack protein, causing it to be destroyed. The proteins become sticky and, therefore, they become attached to each other. The molecules become twisted, that is distorted. Ultimately, this results in organ damage, as well as premature aging.

Experiments have proven that refined sugar damages the arteries, largely through the aforementioned mechanism. Normally, the arteries are elastic. As a result of sugar consumption they become hard or stiff, again, due to cross-linking. Thus, sugar causes these critical organs to age rapidly. Yet, it was Yudkin, former professor emeritus at London's Queen's Hospital, who proved the human connection: as sugar consumption rises, so does the incidence of heart disease. This is true in all societies. The fact is regarding food only sugar has a linear curve. Fats have no major influence, that is the naturally occurring types found in animal and vegetable foods. Repeatedly, Dr. Yudkin pointed out that despite fat intake societies in which there was little or no refined sugar consumption, heart and arterial diseases were/are unknown.

Researchers at Harvard's School of Public Health proved another critical connection: the toxicity of synthetic fats. These fats are found primarily in fast and processed foods. Thus, heavily refined foods are the heart and arteries' doom. By avoiding such foods sudden death from heart disease can be largely curtailed.

Arterial infection: a shocking reality

Doctors, as well as the general public, have always regarded arterial disease as a dietary or toxic issue. The public has been trained to think a certain way. The focus has been on the role of cholesterol in the cause of plugged or hardened arteries. The fact is this substance has been emphasized as the major factor. Cholesterol-rich foods, such as egg yolks, butter, whole milk, cheese, and meat, supposedly cause arterial damage. In humans such a theory has never been proven, in other words, a direct connection has never been documented. On the contrary, it has been thoroughly proven that in indigenous populations, that is where natives regularly eat cholesterol or saturated fat-rich foods, such as the Arctic tribes, the Caucasus Russians, the Turks, the Yemeni Jews, and the Masai, heart disease is virtually unknown. The fat theory for heart disease or that dietary fat alone is the major factor, has been dispelled. There is no known connection between the intake of naturally occurring fats, that is the healthy fats found in food, and heart disease. Yet, there is a definite connection between infectious diseases and heart disease.

This connection was shown by a recent study published in England, which demonstrated that sudden infections, such as an attack of cystitis or bronchitis, increase the risks for heart attacks four-fold. However, this may largely be a red herring. In such infections the treatment is usually antibiotics, which cause fungal invasion. The fungi create sticky masses in the bloodstream, which may lead to clotting and, therefore, heart attack. So, it may not be the infection per se that increases the risk but, rather, the drug therapy. There is an association with long-term antibiotic use and heart attacks. Yet, the fact that human arteries are readily infected is undeniable. Virtually any artery can be infected. In some instances, such as in various forms of vasculitis, the entire arterial tree may become infected. In sepsis, which afflicts some 300,000 Americans yearly, all the arteries are involved. The latter is a systemic infection, which requires aggressive treatment. However, again, in this instance antibiotics fail to cure the disease, in fact, they aggravate it.

It makes sense that arteries can be infected, especially diseased and stiff ones, such as the arteries of atherosclerosis. The word sclerosis, that is scarring, is revealing. Infection is the main cause of scar formation in the body. Entire diseases once thought due to non-infective causes, such as aneurysm, vasculitis, nephritis, temporal arteritis, kidney stones, and arthritis, are now proving to be infective in origin. The infective nature of aortic aneurysm is well established. The fact is germs readily destroy the arterial walls and may largely cause aneurysms. Experiments have proven that if an arterial wall is weakened, germs may enter it, causing its destruction, that is an aneurysm forms. Once such a lesion forms unless the infection is aggressively destroyed, the fatality rate is exceedingly high. Upon the destruction of the infection most aneurysms stabilize, and, as a result, the risk for sudden death declines dramatically.

Again, contrary to popular belief, which mainly blames diet, aneurysms may have their origin in infection. Germs are highly destructive. They can readily damage tissue, including the rather tough arterial walls. True, poor diet ultimately weakens these walls, as well as the immune system, which seeks to protect them. The arterial walls are in a constant state of repair and strain. As mentioned previously as a result of stress, poor nutrition, drug therapy, and toxicity, eventually, they degenerate.

Once the walls are sufficiently weakened the artery balloons out, and an aneurysm develops. Yet, the aggressive damage of the arterial wall starts in infection. This infection often arises from the heart valves, staph and strep being the most common culprits. As a result of the pumping action of the heart the infection can be seeded to virtually any region, including the arteries in the brain. What's more, the entire arterial tree is well supplied with lymphatic vessels. Conceivably, the germs would migrate from the site of infection, potentially infecting the entire arterial system. Yet, the most likely result is gradual spread from the site of origin, for instance, the heart valves to the closely associated aorta. However, these valves are not the true site of the infection. Actually, the infection originates from more remote regions, notably the teeth, gums, sinuses, tonsils, and appendix.

The body makes every conceivable effort to destroy such infections. Yet, often, it is overwhelmed. What's more, these infections are largely due to drug-resistant germs: freaks of nature. The immune system has a difficult time destroying such germs. Furthermore, these germs are located in difficult-to-reach areas such as the linings of the heart valves and inner linings of the arteries. Thus, in order to purge them the body needs help.

This is where wild spice oils are invaluable. Such oils are from edible species of plants, so they can be taken with impunity. In other words, they can be taken in large quantities over a prolonged period—without concern. What's more, the crude, unprocessed wild herb—the OregaMax capsules—has been shown in studies to boost white blood cell function, and it is these cells which scavenge germs from the circulation.

The fact that the arteries are readily infected is indisputable. Remember, dentists are obligated to give antibiotics whenever doing invasive procedures, that is on patients with weak hearts. Yet, such treatment should be routine regardless of the patient's health.

There is an excess of focus on the role of diet in heart disease. Compared to the role of infection diet has minimal impact. True, diet is important. However, it is infection which can cause sudden death. Thus, the role of infection is far more critical than even the role of diet. The fact is to reverse circulatory diseases a change in diet is critical. Yet, this is not the most critical factor.

There is an obvious implication: the focus should be on the infectious sites and their appropriate treatment—this is the crux of the therapy. If the infection is cleansed from the body the entire function of the circulatory system improves. The heart becomes stronger and is less vulnerable to disease. What's more, there is a significant reduction in the likelihood of strokes or blood clots. The risks for massive heat attacks is also significantly reduced. Infections cause the blood to be sticky. When the infections are destroyed, the blood becomes naturally thin. What's more, as a result of successfully eliminating the infection the diet therapy will be more effective.

Infections within the bloodstream, heart, and arteries are highly dangerous. The fact is this is known as blood poisoning. Often the source of such infections is the mouth. The gums, teeth, and surrounding bone are all readily infected. These infections are largely the result of poor hygiene and nutrition. Invasive dentistry is also a major factor. Treatment should be aimed at destroying the infections within this region. The oil of wild oregano (Oreganol P73), as well as the multiple spice OregaDENT, is ideal for this purpose. Both can be regularly rubbed on the gums as preventive medicine. The OregaDENT can also be used as a dentrifice. It has an excellent taste, and, so, it is easier to use regularly. A few drops in salt water makes an excellent gargle. Regular application essentially eliminates swollen gums. This protocol is effective for any kind of gum disease and largely prevents the need for invasive surgery.

Stroke: an infectious disease?

It is well known that surgery can result in blood clots. What's more, it can result in a kind of full body inflammation within the arteries, where the entire blood system suffers from clotting. As a consequence of surgery huge clots can form; massive inflammation of the arteries, heart, kidneys, and even skin can result. The clot obstructs blood flow, leading to further inflammation and swelling. Oxygen can no longer penetrate the tissues. The environment becomes ideal for the spread of germs. The clot becomes septic and, thus, seeds infection. Then, the infection is rapidly transported throughout the bloodstream. Potentially every region of the body becomes infected. Medically, this is known as sepsis and in the extreme, septic shock. At this stage the death rate is high: only four of ten survive.

Post-surgically, every year tens of thousands of individuals suffer from medical catastrophes of frightening proportions. Sepsis strikes seemingly as a routine consequence of surgery. This means that since millions of surgical procedures are performed yearly there are millions of cases of sepsis. Thus, it is important to know the signs and symptoms of this disease. These signs/symptoms include fever, chills, night sweats, joint pain, and internal pain, usually in the abdomen. The body can turn beet red and the skin can be afflicted with nodules and red spots, all secondary to internal clotting and inflammation.

It has been presumed that such a process is due to clotting, in other words, stickiness of the blood, which is secondary to the invasion of surgery. What is rarely recognized is that it is infection that causes this clotting. In other words, without the infection such massive systemic reactions would fail to occur.

Lida Mattman, in her CRC Press-published landmark book, *Cell Wall Deficient Forms: Stealth Pathogens*, has dedicated an entire chapter to this phenomenon, "L-Forms in Thrombi." L-forms are a kind of mutated germ, which are capable of hiding within cells. Thus, such germs usually escape notice, that is by pathologists and microbiologists. They also escape notice of the immune system. Such forms prefer to grow and invade within cells. Thrombi is the medical term for blood clots. She quotes a researcher, who cultured blood clots. He found bizarre forms of bacteria, as well as fungi—the L-forms—within these clots, while people without clots were free of them.

These unique forms of microbes have an apparent preference for blood clot material. Plus, they secrete certain chemicals, which cause a thickening of the arterial walls, while increasing the stickiness of the blood. What's more, they have a genetic defense for survival, that is a system for mutating to their own advantage. One of these bacteria was found to make an enzyme, which splits heparin: the body's natural defense against excessive clotting. The objective of these germs appears to be to thicken the blood in order to create the environment for their further growth. Others produce compounds, which provoke a thickening of the blood and which activate the blood-clotting mechanism, for instance, the platelet-activating powers of certain types of strep.

It has been long known that sepsis, that is wholesale infection of the blood, leads to thickening of the blood and even blood vessel collapse: the so-called intravascular coagulation syndrome. Now there is an explanation for this syndrome: the toxic effects of intracellular bacteria, that is the L-forms.

Is heart attack infectious?

Regarding the so-called syndrome, coronary artery disease, the precursor to heart attacks and heart failure, Mattman also describes a rather ominous statistic: in all cases studied there is evidence of infection. The primary agent is *Chlamydia pneumoniae*, which is a sort of deceptive name. Chlamydia is a bacteria that resembles a fungus. As the name implies it can readily infect the lungs, but it is also capable of infecting any tissue. Notably, it has a high propensity to infect the genitals as well as eyes. Globally, trachoma, a chlamydial infection, is the leading cause of blindness. Yet, this germ is highly aggressive and can infect virtually all organs. Thus, it is no surprise that it is being found in the heart, the heart sac, and arteries. What's more, it has a preference for the coronary arteries, that is the arteries which feed the heart muscle.

The existence of chlamydia gives further proof to the blood clot-infection connection. It was Leinonen, publishing in *Microbiology and Pathogenicity*, who determined that people with clots in their coronary arteries have definite evidence of blood-borne chlamydia infection. Since coronary artery disease afflicts some 33% of the population, obviously, infection by this germ is widespread. The fact is the blood of such individuals is vulnerable to clotting, and this clotting tendency may be directly due to this germ.

Obviously, for health to be restored, as well as for prevention, the germ must be eradicated. This can be accomplished through the intake of high potency spice extracts, particularly the Oreganol, OregaBiotic, and Juice of Oregano. These act as purging agents, eliminating infections from the tissues.

There is further evidence for the germ-heart disease connection. As a consequence of the damage resulting from blood clots disseminated to the heart, fluid accumulates mainly around the heart sac. This fluid may be suctioned and cultured. If this fluid is injected into experimental animals, as well as human cells, chlamydia-like infections occur. This work was performed in the 1970s, long before Chlamydia pneumoniae was known. The fact is this organism was originally cultured from heart tissue, directly related to heart attack and coronary artery disease. Thus, the organism should be re-named *Chlamydia thrombae* (for blood clot formation) or *Chlamydia coronae.* This is because research indicates that this is the key organism, which may be responsible for a wide range of heart and arterial diseases, including arterial inflammation, hardening of the arteries, stroke, sudden blood clots, coronary artery disease, pericarditis, high blood pressure, and even heart attacks.

The evidence for chlamydia's role as the causative agent in heart and arterial disease, and, therefore, hypertension, is vast. Yet, the medical profession has failed to recognize it. However, eventually, it will be forced to recognize it. Consider Altemeir's work in *Annals of Surgery,* 1969, when he accidentally stumbled upon a finding: that sudden or recurring blood clots have an infectious origin. This was followed with a further article, published in *Infectious Diseases,* 1972, in which he claimed that intracellular forms of bacteria are likely the cause of blood clots. Yet, it is well known that clots can travel from distant places in the body, seeding the rest of it with inflammation and infection. Thus, the clot acts as the agent for the spread of infection, in fact, disease.

In England further evidence has been accumulated confirming the chlamydia link. Here, infection of the arterial walls by this germ has been confirmed. Dr. Cook and his group made a dramatic finding: chlamydia, seems to be directly related to the cause of high blood pressure. Some 35% of people with the latter have the infection in their arteries, compared to only 17% of controls. This is sufficient proof of a role played by this germ. Yet, Cook and his colleagues failed to look for the L-Forms, which were likely present in the remainder of the patients.

The infection creates swelling and scarring in the arteries. This causes the heart to work harder, decreasing its pumping powers. As a result the arteries compensate by constricting. This could lead to high blood pressure. Surely, this degree of infection could also lead to the release of bacterial poisons, which could damage sensitive tissues such as the heart muscle and/or its arteries. What's more, these poisons disrupt the function of sensitive nerves, including those which control blood pressure. Plus, the microbial poisons disturb the function of the critical adrenal glands, further compromising the blood pressure mechanism.

Do these bacteria, including chlamydia, infect the blood in general, or do they actually infect the most critical of all organs: the heart muscle itself? It was Arbusine, publishing in the highly orthodox, *American Heart Journal*, who, apparently, provided the proof: the discovery of chlamydia in plaques found in the coronary arteries. This was the ultimate evidence: the germ plays a definite role in heart and arterial disease, since it not only infects the arteries but also infects the very arteries of the heart muscle itself. This is an encouraging finding. This is because it indicates, clearly, that disorders of the heart and arteries are reversible. They can be cured. All that is necessary is to destroy the infection. The inflammation and swelling in the arteries, as well as the scar formation, must be halted. This can largely be achieved by destroying the pathogen. It is the pathogen which causes the inflammation. Thus, to eliminate it the pathogen must be destroyed. As a result, the high blood pressure is reversed.

Yet, the fact that heart disease could be infective should come as no surprise. Consider the opening statements of the book, *Mechanisms of Microbial Disease*, "Infections involving the blood stream, the blood vessels, and the heart tend to be serious, often life threatening." This is where infections begin: in the blood. The blood readily carries infections throughout the body. Any organ can become contaminated, including the heart, the coronary arteries, and the various arteries themselves. For instance, the aorta can become infected, leading to internal damage and, ultimately, aneurysm. The arteries of the brain can become infected, leading to stroke.

Blood is the medium for infection. When microbiologists attempt to grow bacteria, they do so in a medium derived from the blood of various animals: the so-called blood agar. The authors further note that "All the elements of the circulatory system (heart, vessels, blood cells, and plasma) can be subject to infections..." They also note that the number of germs which can infect this system are legion: virtually all known viruses, bacteria, fungi, and parasites. The blood, they write, acts as a "seeding" mechanism, transporting the germs, which may then infect any organ: "As the blood circulates it carries microorganisms from place to place through the body. This can be...harmful to the host."

Of note these microorganisms include fungi, which can cause congealing of the blood. These masses are a kind of fungal balls. Plus, fungi readily infect stagnant blood and blood clots.

It becomes obvious that the orthodox sources make it clear that infection of the blood as a cause of chronic disease is a reality. What's more, as a result of such infections virtually any region of the body, including the heart muscle and arteries, can be damaged. This calls into question the entire modern method for the treatment of heart disease. This is in regards to invasive techniques. This is a method which fails to address the primary cause. Thus, a moratorium should be instituted upon invasive therapies, such as bypass surgery and angioplasty, that is until the role of infection is confirmed.

Surely, such invasive therapies will only worsen the disease, that is by spreading and perpetuating infection. The infection(s) must be cleared chemically, not through aggressive surgical procedures. If the arterial walls are infected and if there is septic matter within them or in the blood, then, invasive procedures will spread it. This may explain the high rate of death following bypass surgery: around 10% or more in certain centers. What's more, the incidence of stroke post-surgically is inordinately high: up to 25% or greater. Mini-strokes are even more common. Typically, loss of mental function occurs in as many as 40% of patients.

Such an aggressive treatment, which fails to address the underlying causes, results in a vast degree of trauma and distress as well as premature death. Furthermore, the financial consequences in terms of actual costs, as well as loss of human efficiency, are beyond count. Thus, the surgery acts to further seed the infection in the bloodstream, causing a high percentage of deaths from sepsis and blood clots. Here, the ideal treatment is to safely kill the germ(s). This causes a reduction in any associated swelling, tissue damage, and inflammation. This should be the future model for the treatment of cardiovascular disease: to ease the damage and trauma while safely destroying the microbes. This will provide a long-term cure, without putting the patient's life at risk.

The degree of danger from invasive treatments is fully documented. If an infection already exists and invasive therapies are applied, a minor infection can be converted into a rampant killer. Schaechter notes in *Mechanisms of Microbial Disease* that today's medical methods are causing blood, as well as organ, infections. Commonly, this is known as blood poisoning or, medically, sepsis. This is a severe type of infection with a high mortality rate: up to 60%. Incredibly, the most severe type, known as septic shock, which routinely kills, is according to Schaechter "a disease of modern medicine; very few cases were reported prior to 1920." He attributes it largely to the extensive use in medicine of invasive techniques, which weaken or damage the body's barriers against infection. He also attributes this to the aggressive use of immunosuppressive drugs, as well as the overuse of antibiotics, the latter being a major cause of systemic fungal infections.

The kidney connection

It has been long known that the kidneys are tied to high blood pressure as well as certain types of arterial and heart diseases. In other words, diseases of the kidneys often result in these conditions. In particular, severe kidney disease, including fulminant infections, result in hypertension. Researchers have attempted to determine the connection, concentrating on certain chemicals produced in the kidney, which control the pressure rate. Yet, the major connection, the role of kidney infection, has rarely if ever been considered. The kidneys are sieves. They act as traps, particularly for germs. Urine is the ideal medium for germ growth. Thus, germs may readily flourish in these organs. The fact is infections of the kidneys are one of the most common conditions afflicting Westerners, with women being particularly vulnerable. If infection becomes established in the kidneys, high blood pressure can result.

A physical or mental disease?

Sodeman, in his book, *Pathologic Physiology: Mechanisms of Disease,* refutes certain myths. He claims that there is no evidence that hypertension is due to nerves. Ruling out mental disease as a primary factor he focuses instead on physical disorders. For instance, he describes the fact that hypertension develops in people with serious kidney infections, the latter being known as pyelonephritis. If the diseased kidney is removed, the hypertension is cured. This clearly demonstrates the infectious link to this disease. This is confirmed by clinical experience. Only rarely is this disease psychological. The fact is in the vast majority of cases it is pathological, that it is a physical disease. Thus, the treatment must correspond.

Sodeman provides further proof for this connection. For years doctors and researchers have concentrated on the kidney connection, but not an infectious one. Every attempt has been made to find a chemical agent, secreted by the kidneys, which accounts for the rise in blood pressure. These attempts have largely failed. Drugs have been created to interfere with the process, which have also failed to produce any cures. Yet, when a diseased kidney, known as an ischemic kidney, that is one with a poor blood and oxygen flow, is transplanted into a healthy animal, the latter develops the disease. This implies that hypertension is transmissible: by a germ or perhaps a group of them. These would likely be fungal forms or, perhaps, cell wall deficient organisms, that is antibiotic resistant mutants. Antibiotic therapy quickly creates mutated bacteria, which flourish in these organs. This is further evidenced by the fact that kidney diseases which are inflammatory, such as nephritis and pyelonephritis, are associated with a rise in blood pressure.

The dental connection

It was Westin Price, DDS, who first delineated the immense role of dental disease in heart and circulatory disorders. He regarded strep as the main culprit causing heart infections. For instance, rheumatic fever, which is a major cause of heart muscle damage, as well as valvular damage, is caused by strep. A high percentage of heart defects in children have infection as their root, particularly strep infection. He then made the dental connection: strep are the main bacteria found in the mouth. Yet, it is likely that fungal forms are equally prominent as causative factors. Fungi are difficult to find and culture. Bacteria are far easier to trace.

Price noted that virtually all dental infections harbor strep. Thus, any invasive therapy, which dislodges such germs, could readily seed the blood: and strep could ultimately infect both the heart and arteries as well as the kidneys. Disorders of all these organs are directly tied to hypertension. He said actual lesions—outright pathology—of the heart and arteries can be caused or worsened by such infections. The diseases he listed, which may be related to dental infections, include inflammation of the heart muscle, inflammation of the heart muscle sac (pericarditis), heart block, aortic disease, high blood pressure, hardening of the arteries, blood clots, anemia, Raynaud's disease, even diabetes.

Note the emphasis on infections of the heart valves, which are thoroughly connected to dental disease. This is why doctors give antibiotics to anyone with heart valve defects, that is in order to prevent seeding the infection. Yet, Price described other sources for the infection, for instance, the tonsils. It is known that the organs can be chemically infected by a wide range of germs, including mutated bacteria, molds, and fungi. In other words, there may be a number of pathogens, which attack the circulatory system and/or kidneys. The sinuses could be an additional source, that is as a pocket of infection. The point is that in the cases of a high percentage of heart or arterial disease patients, including those with high blood pressure, a known or unknown pocket of infection exists, which continuously seeds germs into the bloodstream.

As mentioned previously the linings of arteries in people with heart disease, hardening of the arteries, and high blood pressure appear abnormal and are frequently filled with noxious tissue. They have the appearance of degeneration due to toxic insults. The most likely source of these insults are germs.

The close relationship between dental infections and kidney disease has been thoroughly documented. Price quotes cases in which the urine was constantly contaminated with pus and germs and which after extracting the suspect teeth became clear. The condition "entirely disappeared" after the removal of all infected teeth.

The scope of this dilemma is vast. Could it be that a high percentage of individuals suffering from chronic or recurrent kidney and/or bladder disorders, in fact, have their teeth to blame? Price noted that it was the root-filled teeth that were the primary culprits: in other words fillings and root canals. The fillings trap the sepsis within the teeth, which must find an outlet. That outlet is the blood and lymph, which carry the germs and contaminants to the internal organs, notably the heart muscle, heart valves, and kidneys. The brain is also readily contaminated by this sepsis, which may account for a wide range of neurological and mental diseases, including, incredibly, Alzheimer's disease, Parkinson's disease, ALS, stroke, and multiple sclerosis.

Infections in the teeth have a direct and negative effect upon the nervous system as well as the muscles and joints. The fact is in an individual suffering from disorders of the nerves, brain, muscles, tendons, and/or joints, a thorough dental history must be taken, as is demonstrated by the following.

CASE HISTORY:

Mr. P., a 30-year-old hair dresser, complained of a stiff neck, which for him was unusual. Massage failed to relieve it. He never before had such a problem but merely attributed it to bending over while cutting hair. A complete history was taken. A month prior to developing the stiff neck he suffered a toothache on the same side as his neck pain. A root canal was performed. Within two weeks he became noticeably tired, while also developing the pain. Clearly, the dental surgery was directly connected to his decline in health. Upon taking the wild oregano oil (P73) he improved noticeably, with greater energy and a reduction in the pain.

It becomes obvious that septic teeth are a major cause of disease. However, people rarely make the connection. For the disease burden to be eased the teeth must be treated, either with antiseptics or through extraction. What's more, the blood must be cleansed of all infection, that is through the intake of natural germicides. Mere dental cleaning alone will fail to solve it, since the infections are deep within the tissues. Thus, only a germ-killing approach or removal of the offending tissue will prove effective.

The toxins produced in septic teeth have great ill effects upon the internal organs, with the heart, arteries, brain, and kidneys being the most susceptible. It is these organs which are primarily involved in hypertension. Repeatedly, Price has shown the danger of infected teeth. Taking either parts of the crushed teeth or mere washings thereof, he injected animals with the contaminants: in all cases the rabbits developed severe disease, and usually within 48 hours. Massive disease, including clots, hemorrhage, and cellular death, was confirmed in the muscles, tendons, and joints. The internal organs were fatally damaged.

This demonstrates the incredible degree of toxicity of bacterial, as well as fungal, toxins. The fact is such toxins are produced by these organisms in a kind of self-defense. The toxins are meant to kill other bacteria. Thus, they are the germs' self-defense. However, in sufficient quantity they can be deadly to other creatures, particularly rabbits and other small mammals. They are also deadly to humans, usually through a slow death, that is the decay of chronic disease.

Bacterial poisons are known to cause serious disease as well as sudden death. It is no surprise that they are implicated in high blood pressure. Price, in his book, *Dental Infections and Degenerative Diseases*, Volume II, describes two clinical cases directly tied to septic teeth. The most compelling one is as follows: a woman aged forty-seven had strikingly high blood pressure, the systolic, as well as diastolic, measuring over 200. She suffered from marked pain, a kind of distress in the head, "was almost incapacitated, and the symptoms were quite alarming." Doctors had given up on her. X-ray documented severe inflammation in the jaw bone near the molars.

The suspected tooth and the two surrounding it were extracted; the bone was scraped of all necrotic material. As a result, "her blood pressure, which had been high for over a year, rapidly descended to 125 and has remained...normal ever since." Price also described that "her physical condition returned completely to normal." Interestingly, he commented, a few years prior to the onset of the high blood pressure she suffered an abdominal attack due to a large ovarian cyst. Price's conclusion: the cyst was directly tied to the septic tooth. Thus, the rotting tooth, as well as the necrotic bone surrounding it, had effectively poisoned the woman's entire system, particularly the endocrine glands, fully causing systemic disease. In such rotting tissue in addition to bacteria numerous fungal forms flourished.

Price dedicated an entire chapter to the role of dental infections in heart and arterial diseases, providing numerous case histories of this connection. In his animal studies he thoroughly proved that septic discharge from the teeth directly affects the blood status, poisoning the blood cells as well as the bone marrow. This can lead to a thickening of the blood, increasing the risk for systemic disease. If the sepsis remains untreated or if it worsens, the thickening can develop uncontrollably, resulting in blood clots. What is certain is that septic discharge from the teeth causes inflammation within the bloodstream as well as the arterial walls. Price never proved a direct connection, that is to blood clots, but he did prove that the septic secretions from the teeth of people with blood clots causes massive arterial inflammation.

This inflammation can extend to the heart. This can result in a condition known as cardiomyopathy. Here, the entire heart muscle becomes swollen and inflamed. Untreated, the muscle can degenerate, leading to sudden death. Price describes a patient whose heart was enlarged and inflamed and who also had high blood pressure. The patient suffered from a sensation of extreme tightness in his head and symptoms previously diagnosed as stomach trouble. Careful dental evaluation finally discovered the problem: septic molars. Interestingly, his blood calcium was low, as was his red and white count. The low blood calcium is a sign of bone loss, perhaps also from the teeth and dental bones. The putrefying material around his molars was cultured. Then, it was injected into two rabbits. Within 12 hours one rabbit died of massive arterial collapse. Tiny hemorrhages were found throughout the rabbit's muscles. The bacterial toxins were so powerful that they completely overwhelmed the animal's immune system. The heart muscle of this rabbit was large and flabby, showing evidence of direct toxic damage.

Price concluded that due to the degree of toxicity radical treatment was required. Incredibly, after the extraction of the toxic teeth and the intake of a calcium-rich diet (natural buttermilk), along with calcium supplements, the patient's blood calcium returned to normal. The health of the patient improved dramatically to such a degree that he stated "he had not felt so well in years." His appetite improved and his white count rose to normal. In other words, the person's entire body began functioning normally, whereas he had been in a dire state prior. Price proved that toxic infection disrupts virtually all key body functions and that a rapid cure results, that is when such infections are eradicated.

In the past the only treatment available was tooth extraction, perhaps combined with the use of salt water irrigations. However, now, although extractions still play a role, it is no longer necessary to extract all the sick teeth. Natural antiseptics have solved that. There are a number of natural oils, which can be applied to the teeth and which can be taken internally to deal with the sepsis. Such a treatment will also eliminate the systemic symptoms, that is the high blood pressure, arthritis, heart stress, and inflammation, which are associated with such infections.

Proper hygiene is also essential. Yet, there are times when pulling the teeth is required. What's more, the individual must deal with the mechanical consequences, that is how to safely correct the anatomical defect without worsening the problem. The point is simple. Price proved that hypertension can be cured: quickly. Incredibly, by treating the cause he reversed the disease in as little as a few days. The same can happen today, perhaps without tooth extraction. This is through the aggressive use of antiseptic oils, notably the Oreganol and the OregaDENT multiple spice formula. These two oils formulas are best suited for the oral cavity. Plus, since they are from edible spices they may be taken internally with impunity. There are no side effects to such oils, rather, only benefits.

The OregaDENT is a special combination of oils, which rapidly kill oral pathogens. It is ideal for applying to gums and teeth. It may also be added to mouthwashes and/or rubbed on floss. There is also the OregaSpray which can be used as a dental or throat spray. To order OregaDENT check high quality health food retailers or call 1-800-243-5242.

The data proving the dental connection is compelling. As described in *Family Practice News*, February 2001, Zolu demonstrated an ominous finding: gum disease leads to heart attacks. He discovered a three-fold greater risk for heart attacks in people with severe gum disease than in those with relatively normal gums. The conclusion of the researchers is that gum disease is a far more significant risk factor than any other issue, including high cholesterol, age, sex, alcohol consumption, and even smoking.

Poor dental hygiene is disastrous. This threatens all age groups. In adults and the elderly it can result in cardiovascular disease. In children the consequences can be diabetes and kidney disease. There is also a connection in pregnant mothers. This is through the syndrome known as eclampsia, in which pregnant women develop fluid retention as well as high blood pressure, and this threatens the health of both the mother and fetus. As published in *Obstetrics and Gynecology* high blood pressure, as well as premature birth, are directly correlated with gum disease, that is chronic infection of the gums and tooth sockets. Here, researchers correlate the production by bacteria of endotoxins, which are potent circulatory and cellular poisons. This, they believe, is the source of the toxemia of pregnancy. Such toxins damage the kidneys, leading to inflammation, protein loss in the urine, and fluid retention. Thus, if the infection is cleared, the toxemia will disappear, as will the swelling and kidney dysfunction. It was researchers at the University of North Carolina, who took this a degree further. In a five year study of 850 women investigators determined that gum and tooth disease not only negatively affect pregnant mothers but also "adversely affect babies in wombs." Born early the babies are too small, in fact, septic. What's more, as further evidence of an infectious connection they suffered from an increased risk of heart defects.

The gums are extensively supplied by blood vessels. In the event of periodontal infection the connection is obvious. Pockets, sores, wounds, and holes in the mouth are ready outlets for germs entering the bloodstream. As described on the Web site for the American Academy of General Dentistry even normal gum treatment, mere brushing and flossing, can cause sepsis. Imagine the consequence of aggressive dentistry: gum surgery, root canals, fillings, implants, and crowns. All such procedures disseminate infection.

If the infection is significant, germs may enter the arterial walls or, perhaps, the lining of the heart. Here, they gain a sort of residence, causing chronic infection. This leads to inflammation and, ultimately, scarring. This is the classic hardening of the arteries and/or scarring or prolapse of the heart valves.

Evidence exists that even tumor-like lesions develop on the arterial lining. When such tumors are scraped and the cells viewed, infection may be seen. The culprits: Chlamydia and herpes. The fact is both these germs are associated with scarring of the arterial walls and in the case of herpes scarring of the heart valves. Regarding the latter a type of "malignant" high blood pressure has been associated with it, that is pulmonary hypertension.

Clearly, periodontal disease is related to heart disease. Sick, diseased gums lead to damaged and diseased arteries. It is not through the mechanism that most people might think, that is direct infection of the heart. Rather, it is through a kind of toxic mechanism, where the microbial poisons contaminate the entire body and the entire circulatory system. This places great pressure on the heart. In fact, the heart muscle may be intoxicated by such poisons. What's more, bacteria, as well as other germs, including fungi and parasites, cause a sticky condition of the blood, which also greatly strains the heart. These germs cause lumps, which the body has difficulty dissolving. Plus, bacteria produce toxins which congeal the blood. Fungi are even more aggressive in this regard, producing a wide range of potent chemicals known as mycotoxins. Such toxins rapidly destabilize the circulatory system, leading to clot formation, even heart attack and stroke.

The heart must work additionally to pump blood through such clumps. The clumps are living infective balls, spreading germs throughout the body. When the clumps attach to the arterial walls, damage occurs. Yet, the greatest damage occurs when these clumps penetrate the smaller arteries—the microscopic ones, which supply the arteries themselves. The germ-infested clumps enter directly into the inner linings of the artery walls. This leads to a thickening and, ultimately, scarring. These are known as plaques. To help heal the microbe-induced damage the body lays down cholesterol, which is a sealant, literally a wax. This is an attempt by the body to smooth the roughened surface created by infections.

All this places great stress upon the heart muscle. This explains the findings of the Italian researchers, Fabio and his group, who found that people with gum disease have a much higher incidence of heart damage than those with normal gums. In particular, he found that gum disease is directly correlated with enlargement of the heart muscle component known as the left ventricle. As the degree of infection in the gums rose, so did the degree of heart muscle damage. Yet, other research points to disease of the arteries as a factor, seemingly unrelated to the heart. It was researchers from the University of Colorado, publishing in the *New England Journal of Medicine*, who showed that in the case of pulmonary hypertension there is an ominous finding: herpes-like viruses infecting the blood vessels of the lungs. These viruses inflame the linings of the blood vessels, causing their linings to thicken. Again, this places undue pressure on the heart, potentially leading to heart failure. Thus, many cases of cardiac collapse may be due to hidden infection, particularly if weakened lungs are involved. Incredibly, the herpes virus may also be found in the brain, where it readily causes brain damage and/or stroke. Such infections must be purged from the body in order to halt the risk for cardiovascular disorders and/or sudden death. Thus, both chlamydia and herpes are involved in circulatory damage.

The nutritional connection to dental disease is undeniable. The teeth and gums are vital organs. They require nourishment.

What's more, they are readily damaged by deficient diet. In fact, this organ system is exceedingly vulnerable to vile dietary practices. It was again Westin Price who proved the connection showing that vitamin/mineral deficiency is a major factor in dental and gum diseases. As described by James Rorty in *Tomorrow's Food,* in his studies on primitive societies Price clearly showed that after adopting a Western diet the teeth of these people degenerated with "astonishing rapidity". In their native world, such people never developed high blood pressure nor heart disease. Yet, shortly after adopting this degenerative diet both diseases arose. The famous British investigator, Russell Bunting, confirmed this, noting that the incidence of dental disease in primitives was exceedingly low, while the incidence in people consuming the Western, that is processed food, diet was exceedingly high: some 10% compared to 90%. In other words, 9 of 10 Westerners have diseased oral cavities, while only about 1 of 10 primitives do so.

When primitives adopt the Western diet, rapidly, they assume the same dire percentage as in Westerners. What's more, correspondingly, they develop heart disease and hypertension at the same rate as Westerners. This creates a critical issue: is it possible that a person can remain impervious to heart disease and/or hypertension, that is as long as his or her dental health is in ideal condition? This is a premise worth investigating.

The mechanisms of dental infections are of interest. The enamel can break down, and germs may invade either from the top or the side of the tooth. Once in the tooth it festers, producing pus and poisons. The infection may also fester within pockets, which develop along the teeth. There may also develop a generalized infection within the gum tissue, which can lead to leakage into the general circulation. Germs love to hide. So, if they penetrate into the teeth, they are in a sense sequestered from the immune system. From here they may burrow into the jaw bone, where they cause a bone infection known as osteomyelitis. The infection may become severe enough to cause bone death, known as necrosis.

Fischer, in his book, *Death and Dentistry*, rejects the concept of cavities. He claims that the teeth are boney extensions, so any infection is a form of bone infection. Thus, what are now known as cavities, according to Fischer's definition, are, in fact, pockets of osteomyelitis, that is fulminant infections of the bone. This potentially emphasizes the dire consequences of aggressive dental procedures: the spread of infection deep into the bone. The fact is any direct invasion of the teeth will result in bone infection.

The teeth cannot be infected without corresponding involvement of the underlying bone, that is the bones of the jaw and face. What's more, aggressive dentistry, that is deep drilling, will assuredly result in deep-seated bone infections. Thus, virtually anyone who has undergone aggressive dental drilling has at least a low grade bone infection. Fischer, former professor of physiology at the Joseph Eichber Laboratory, University of Cincinnati, made a revolutionary observation. In his book, *Death and Dentistry*, he begins by considering the starting point which all dentists, as well as patients, understand: decay. This, he notes, is found in the top of the tooth going downward and possibly at its neck. He first raises the question, that is "what is this so-called decay? The dentist terms it caries. Pathologically it is a spot of dead bone, more technically a necrosis. We add at once that *invariably* it is infected."

Yet, this infection fails to remain in the teeth/bones. Particularly, through invasive dentistry it is spread directly into the bloodstream. There is a more indirect path: through tiny vessels, which function to carry wastes from the tissues, that is the lymph vessels. Ultimately, all lymph, which is a kind of protein-rich or milky fluid, dumps into the bloodstream, essentially directly above the heart. The germs are then carried by the blood through the rest of the body. This is how infection is spread, because every organ in the body is supplied by blood vessels.

It is well known that the heart muscle has its own arteries, that is the coronary arteries. What is little known is that each artery has its own blood vessels, tiny tubes known as the *vasa vasorum*. Each artery is surrounded by such blood vessels, which directly feed the arterial walls, including the walls of the coronary arteries. Again, it was Fischer who in early research proved that infection develops within the circulatory organs by direct seeding of the infection through the arteries, that is the vasa vasorum, which directly supply blood to all arteries, including the coronary arteries. This makes sense: germs from the teeth enter the bloodstream, where they cause coagulation, that is blood clots. These are not usually huge clots, rather, they are micro-clots. These micro-clots spread throughout the circulatory system and are carried even into the tiniest blood vessels, including those which surround the arteries.

In essence the arteries deliver the germ-contaminated clots directly into the arterial wall, where they lodge. This blocks the flow of blood to the arteries, and, thus, these tissues become oxygen-starved. This is the beginning of atherosclerosis, that is hardening of the arteries. Fischer has provided pictures as proof: actual germs arising from the mouth, which are lodged into the arterial wall, not the walls inside the blood vessel lumen but, rather, from the outside in: from the outer blood supply. This proves that the infection is transmitted by the blood supply of the organ itself.

This is important, because it means that the key to reversing heart disease is to kill any infection in the blood itself or within the source of the infection, for instance, septic teeth, tonsils, sinuses, colon, adenoids, bones, etc. Thus, for a person to be cured of any serious circulatory disease the source(s) of chronic infection, which seeds into the blood, must be eradicated. Then, the blood itself must be purged of any remaining infection. This is achieved through spice oil extracts, which are fully capable of destroying both local and systemic infections. Their immense power in destroying infections and, therefore, reversing disease is demonstrated by the following:

CASE HISTORY:

Mr. C., a 60-year-old man, suddenly developed breast cancer. The lesion became so severe that his nipple fell off. His only other major health problem was relatively severe high blood pressure, about 200/120. He had a history of gum disease, but no one considered this. Opting for a more natural approach, while refusing chemotherapy, he took the oil of wild oregano (Oreganol P73) as well as the juice of wild oregano. Incredibly, within a month the cancerous lesion disappeared. What's more, his blood pressure dropped dramatically in merely a month to 140/90. With a history of both a kind of septic breast cancer and gum disease, surely infection was at the root of his high blood pressure. What's more, since diseased gums are correlated with cancer the entire disorder could be related directly to infection: in the teeth and gums.

Regarding the modern view of the disease, Fischer makes an interesting comment. He admits that modern medicine regards common diseases, such as heart disease and high blood pressure, as "degenerative." In other words, the possibility that these are infective is never considered. The medical profession, he claims, places such diseases in their own categories attempting to discover a biological or chemical link or perhaps a stress-related cause. There is also emphasis on diet, including fat and cholesterol as well as salt reduction. Yet, according to Fischer bacterial (or other microbial) plugs are the key factors which are rarely if ever addressed. Such plugs, rather, clots, occlude the flow of blood to the arteries, causing a phenomenon known as infarction. The latter is defined as cell death due to a lack of blood flow and/or oxygen.

The cell death is ideal for the germs: now they can readily invade, further destroying the tissue. This is what germs do best, that is attack and invade weakened and/or dead tissues. Anyone who has closely examined the arteries of atherosclerotic victims knows that there is cell death throughout the arterial walls. Again, while the emphasis is continually upon diet, alcohol consumption, commercial salt excess, stress, emotional distress, and similar factors, "microorganisms have been caught in the nutritive capillaries" of the arteries. In other words, disease-causing germs have been discovered in the blood supply to diseased arteries as well as within the arterial wall itself. Yet, in the medical approach to disease this key factor is ignored.

All scientists agree that in hypertension and heart disease the arteries are injured. All concede that they are inflamed. Fisher merely claims that it is the germs which are the main cause of such injury and inflammation—germs, which are found precisely in the injured tissue—and that all other factors are secondary. Thus, a vast range of cardiovascular diseases, including vasculitis, arteritis, blood clots, hardening of the arteries, temporal arteritis, hypertension, heart attacks, heart failure, heart valve disorders, and even hemorrhoids, as well as varicose veins, may be directly attributed to infection.

The early German researcher, Huebner, found that in known infections, in this case, syphilis, hardening of the arteries occurred. The interesting issue is that such hardening occurred in the site of infection, in this case, syphilis of the brain. Like Fisher he determined through careful examination that the infection was spread through the microcirculation, that is the tiny blood vessels, which supply the arteries of the brain. He too observed that these tiny vessels, known medically as arterioles and capillaries, became plugged by bacterial clots. Now it is known that such clots may also be fungal, even parasitic. In fact, fungi are a major cause of obstructive clots.

Fischer describes numerous case histories of people, whose blood pressure was decreased as a result of anti-infection regimens. Such regimens were largely based upon dental therapy, that is the removal of any diseased teeth or tissue followed by the use of antiseptics, notably iodine and salt water. As a result of this treatment in the majority of the cases the high blood pressure was significantly reduced.

Today, the methods of treatment are more sophisticated. Oil of wild oregano is far superior to iodine. Salt water infusions, perhaps combined with vinegar, may still be applied. There are many excellent preventive-minded dentists, who can determine the necessity of tooth extraction. There are also herbal and food supplement programs, which help cleanse the tissues of toxins, while aiding in the rebuilding of cells. In addition, certain nutrients have been proven to strengthen the gums and the teeth, preventing infectious degeneration. For instance, there is the unprocessed wild oregano capsules—the OregaMax—which are rich in naturally occurring, bone building calcium and phosphorous. The regular intake of this supplement leads to bone deposition, while strengthening gum tissue. There is also the wild spice spray, the OregaSpray, as well as the OregaDENT. Thus, today, the results are even more superior than they were in Fischer's time, that is the 1930s.

The fact that heart and arterial disorders could be due to infection was known even earlier: in the late 1800s. This was when there was great research regarding the role of germs in heart and arterial diseases. From about 1875 until the 1940s hundreds of medical textbooks were produced delineating an infectious role. Consider Salinger's *Modern Medicine*, published in 1900. In this book the role of infection as a cause of heart and arterial damage is clearly described. For instance, according to Salinger regarding disease of the heart valves, including mitral valve prolapse, "the lining of the valves" is infected and even infective "ulcers" may form. "Abscesses of the myocardium may form," which can lead to "rupture," that is massive heart attack.

The term rupture is highly significant. This can only be caused by infection, which creates scarring of the valves and, thus, causes them to split upon the pressure of the pumping of the heart. This is precisely what happened to one patient, Mr. M., whose doctor told him that his heart attack was caused by a sudden rupture of his heart valves (see page 46). Incredibly, according to Salinger "various micro-organisms and their toxins...are often present in the blood." So, heart, heart valvular, and arterial diseases may not be due to a single germ but, instead, multiple germs. Even without the sophistication of today's labs, Salinger determined that the toxins produced by the germs are largely the cause of these diseases.

Even in this early era rather bizarre groups of germs were proven to cause cardiovascular infections, including oral strep, the measles virus, gonorrhea, syphilis, the typhoid bacillus, pneumococcus, and the malarial parasite. However, then the role of fungi as a cause of micro-clots was unknown. The fact is disease of the heart valves may be caused by the aforementioned germs, as well as, more recently, proven perpetrators—black mold, *Candida albicans*, the fungus of histoplasmosis, E. coli, and Listeria.

Yet, apparently, the poisons produced by germs are equally devastating to the circulatory system as the germs themselves. This is demonstrated by dental research. Again, it was Price who proved that merely injecting the septic wastes from a diseased tooth, that is a tooth, which was loaded with microbial toxins, caused sudden death in experimental animals. Again, this demonstrates the extreme toxicity of microbial poisons of dental origin on the human organs.

The poisons placed by dentists in the mouth are equally vile. It was Hal Huggins, DDS, M.S. who first revealed it. An orthodox dentist for over 40 years he abandoned the standard approach due to concerns of toxicity.

Dr. Huggins has made people aware of the dangers of both root canals and dental amalgam. He describes thousands of cases of people who were poisoned, even killed, by orthodox dentistry. A dear friend, he notes, a healthy doctor, died suddenly. The cause: extreme gum scraping, which disseminated a fatal sepsis. According to Dr. Huggins the victim spent two hours having his gums scraped, which were severely inflamed. The dentist earned major income, yet within two days the patient was dead. This is why according to Dr. Huggins if aggressive dentistry was curbed the heart disease and high blood pressure epidemic would be reversed. Regarding high blood pressure he notes, "How many cases of high blood pressure do we see who do not have root canals? Less than 10%." More on this dentist's research can be found on his 150 page Web site, www.drhuggins.com.

Serious infections of the heart and arteries cannot be regarded as uncommon. This is particularly true of hospitalized patients, as well as individuals, who develop severe or sudden illnesses, particularly severe dental infections, blood poisoning, meningitis, encephalitis, and pneumonia. In any of these conditions heart and heart valve infections could be expected. There may not be obvious cardiac symptoms. Rather, this may be manifested by generalized fatigue, intolerance to exercise, and weakness. Stiffness of the joints, including the spinal column and neck, are common. There may also be some mild shortness of breath upon exertion. Vague or constant chest pain may also occur, which is usually diagnosed as stress or anxiety. Usually, the cause is never determined.

Surgery: major risk factor

It is well known that surgery spreads infection. This is no condemnation of the procedure. There are times when surgery is necessary. However, regardless of the skill of the surgeon any invasive procedure can lead to infection.

The most minor injury can lead to systemic infection. Once the barriers are broken the body is vulnerable. There are many warnings regarding the signs and symptoms of blood poisoning: red streaks, fever, chills, and racing heart. How many people do you know, perhaps yourself, your children, or friends, who have developed some form of blood poisoning after an injury or surgery?

According to the *Journal of the American Medical Association* in hospitals blood poisoning, known medically as sepsis, is an epidemic. The Journal describes the fact that sepsis claims the lives of some 250,000 Americans, an ominous statistic. The majority of these deaths occur post-surgically. In other words, the infections developed as a consequence of surgery, and to halt them nothing can be done. Or, there was a minor injury, which was treated in a hospital or doctor's office, and it became septic, leading to uncontrollable infection. Thus, people die unmerciful deaths merely as a result of minor wounds, like a scrape or cut. Imagine the risks of major abdominal, dental, or cardiac surgery. The fact is the risks are vast.

This demonstrates a simple fact: there is no reason to undergo surgery, that is unless absolutely necessary. The risks for systemic infection are too great, particularly today. Endocarditis, that is infection of the heart valves, is merely one of these infections. Thus, heart disease may have its origin in surgery, where germs are disseminated in the blood and where they ultimately infect the heart, heart valves, and/or arteries. Anyone with heart- or arterial-related symptoms must be evaluated for surgical/dental history. This is also true of people with hypertension, vasculitis, arteritis, varicose veins, and stroke. In these diseases the possibility for a systemic infection exists, which creates inflammation and cell damage—and which may lead to the creation of septic clots—all due to surgically-induced infection. Whenever evaluating circulatory disease this is one of the most critical factors to consider.

In hospitals sepsis is rampant, and the incidence is rising dramatically every year. What's more, the majority of infections involve drug-resistant organisms. Incredibly, the development of post-surgical infections has become virtually routine. Ominously, such infections are virtually expected, that is in those who undergo a significant surgery, such as heart bypass, gallbladder or appendix removal, hysterectomy, colon resection, or similar major procedures, the development of secondary infections is automatic. What's more, antibiotics will fail to halt it.

Kidney infections: the missing link?

The role of kidney, as well as bladder, infections in the cause of high blood pressure is immense. The fact is regarding acute hypertensive crises kidney infections play a prominent role. The claim for the involvement of the kidneys in high blood pressure is nothing new. However, here a new means of understanding it is proposed. This is the fact high blood pressure is caused not only from sudden or toxic infections but also because of chronic or smoldering infections, which fail to be addressed medically. There is a plethora of evidence for this. Let us review it systematically.

The kidneys act as a trap. One of the things they trap are germs. If the germs cannot be properly cleared by the immune system, infection gains a foothold. This may result in chronic infection of the kidneys, as well as bladder, predisposing to hypertension. The infection causes the release of certain chemicals, which raise blood pressure. Plus, again, bacterial, as well as fungal, clots are released, which damage blood vessels throughout the body.

Germs from the mouth are commonly found in the kidneys. Recall that strep infection is a serious concern regarding these organs. In the mouth strep is the most prolific organism. Dentists are keenly aware of the risk. Untold thousands of cases of potentially fatal strep infections of the kidneys have arisen from invasive dentistry. That is why dentists are obligated in the event of invasive surgery to recommend antibiotics, that is for those who are vulnerable to kidney infections. Yet, there is no guarantee that in healthy individuals there is any exemption. The mere filling of cavities can seed infections into the kidney. Incredibly, so can vigorous brushing and flossing. The fact is anyone who suffers from kidney and/or bladder ailments must have their dental status assessed. Are such individuals victims of root canals and/or multiple fillings or perhaps some other highly invasive procedure? All such facts must be ascertained, that is for the appropriate cure to be achieved. Regarding germ protection for dental procedures the oil of wild oregano, as well as the more tasty spice mixture, that is the OregaDENT, are particularly effective. The fact is such spice oils are more effective, as well as more safe, than antibiotics.

Vaccines: damage beyond comprehension

Vaccines introduce a wide range of toxins in the body, including harsh chemicals, solvents, chemical preservatives, heavy metals, emulsifiers, detergents, and a varying 'soup' of microbes. It is a false concept that vaccines are sterile. They cannot be. This is because they are created in an animal environment—on animal cells and within animal fluids—plus they represent the specific attempt to grow and harvest microbes for injection into the body. Thus, regardless of the procedure used for sterilization contamination is inevitable. What's more, in the majority of vaccines the sterilization techniques are incomplete. Inevitably, germs will escape, particularly today with the vast panorama of drug- and chemical-resistant organisms. There are even germs, which are resistant to chlorine. Thus, the concept of the sterilization of vaccines is a fraud.

Researchers in the government have proven a simple fact: the original vaccines given during the height of the vaccine industry's growth, such as the oral (sugar cube) polio vaccine, were extensively contaminated. That contamination was transferred to humans and is responsible for the onset of a variety of diseases. Michelle Carbone, Ph.D., has documented a bizarre, in fact, frightening finding: virus-infected tumors of the brain and lungs. The source of the virus: contaminated oral polio vaccines from the 1950s and 60s. The contaminant is a monkey virus, the so-called Simian Virus 40. This contamination is due to the fact that the original vaccine was grown on monkey kidney cells harvested from African and, particularly Indian, monkeys, including chimpanzees.

What a vile deed it was, that is to contaminate people all over the world, particularly Americans and Canadians, with monkey viruses. Yet, incredibly, the people who did so won Nobel Prizes: for corrupting the human race? This vile act has caused an insurmountable degree of disease and devastation as well as an untold number of premature deaths. The fact is even today people are developing tumors secondary to these viruses. What's more, a vast degree of ill health is occurring, that is those chronic degenerative diseases for which there are no diagnoses or cures: these are likely the result of the monkey virus contamination, which occurred particularly in anyone who received such vaccines from the mid-1950s through 60s. The residues of these viruses must be purged from the body. This is achieved through the wild oregano protocol. This protocol consists of the intake of the juice of wild oregano, the edible (i.e. P73) oil of wild oregano, and the OregaBiotic multiple spice capsule. This is a triple action protocol for eradicating deep seated and hidden infections. For best results be sure to use all three medicines. The protocol is as follows:

- Juice: one or more ounces twice daily
- Oil of Oreganol (P73): a dropperful twice daily
- OregaBiotic (garlic, onion, oregano, allspice oil formula)
- OregaDENT (clove, cinnamon, and P73 oregano oil formula)
- Health-Bac: 1/2 tsp. or more at bedtime in warm water

The oil alone is certainly germicidal. However, the OregaBiotic is exceptionally powerful and is a great adjunct for the eradication of deep-seated infections. The protocol should be followed for a minimum of 90 days, or, preferably, 120 days. For tough or extreme cases follow this for a minimum of six months, then, follow a maintenance program of one-half the aforementioned. There is a word of caution. With such high doses there might be an initial rise in blood pressure. However, remain vigilant. Eventually, in fact, rather quickly, the blood pressure will normalize, in fact, be reduced.

One way to minimize this is to consume plenty of natural bacteria in the form of yogurt, quark, kefir as well as healthy bacterial supplements. Yet, if it does rise, the only reason for this is that wild oregano improves the pumping power of the heart. To help prevent such an initial rise take the crude red grape, that is the Resvital, four capsules twice daily. This helps create elasticity in the arteries, which due to the many years of abuse and drug therapy, have become stiffened. The combination of the crude red sour grape plus the P73 wild oregano is even superior to the oregano alone in causing a reduction of blood pressure. The oral polio vaccine is far from the only fully contaminated vaccine. Evidence exists that virtually all modern vaccines are toxic, incredibly, some are even infected with various monkey viruses, including SV40. Other contaminants include tubercular-like germs, syphilitic germs, mycoplasmas, fungi, molds, and various encephalitis viruses, as well as bizarre genetically engineered germs. People who receive modern vaccines, including the flu vaccine, should undergo the aforementioned protocol.

The glands may be damaged by vaccines, particularly the adrenals and the thyroid. Support may also be needed here. For the adrenals take Royal Power, four capsules daily. For the thyroid take Thyroset, three capsules twice daily. There is also the Royal Oil, which may be taken under the tongue. For tough cases this should also be taken, about a half teaspoon twice daily.

Acute high blood pressure attacks: the so-called hypertensive emergencies

Hypertensive emergencies are avoidable. This is because the vast majority of these are caused by toxic stress and/or infection. If the stress is dealt with and the toxins are neutralized, no emergency need occur. What's more, as is mentioned throughout this book, the infection, which is the root of the crisis, can be cleansed, that is before an emergency develops.

It is critical to avoid such an emergency. The death rate from hypertensive crisis is high. So is the complication rate: stroke, heart failure, systemic infection, and heart attack. The crisis commonly occurs in pregnant women and can result in premature labor, premature birth, infant death, and abortion. What is certain is that in any case of hypertensive crisis the underlying infection must be treated. In hospitals if this approach were taken, uncountable complications, as well as premature death, could be aborted. Only nutritional support, herbal medicine, nerve/muscle relaxation, stress management, and similar therapies can cure such crises. The drugs used for this crisis are highly dangerous, in fact, deadly. For information on the natural treatment for hypertensive crisis see Appendix A.

Heart valve infections: modern plague

Medically, infection of the heart valves is known as endocarditis. This is an infection of the special lining within the heart known as the endocardium. Today, this disorder is a severe epidemic, although in general physicians fail to realize its scope. Every year in North American millions of cases of this disorder are missed by physicians. For patients this could prove fatal.

In medicine the possibility of a heart infection is often regarded as remote. Yet, it was S. Rahimtoola, in *Infective Endocarditis*, who made it clear that all parts of the heart tissue are subject to infection. One of the most common of these is the heart valves.

Infective endocarditis is a condition afflicting the inner lining of the heart, that is the lining from which blood is pumped. There are two main types of endocarditis. First, there is the sudden type, which strikes without warning. This is known as acute endocarditis, and it has a high death rate: some 60%. If this severe form of the infection is contracted, there is no drug which will cure it. In fact, the 60% fatality rate is despite the use of antibiotics. The other type is chronic. In the acute type staph and strep, along with pneumococcus, are the primary culprits. Recently, the yeast, *Candida albicans*, has been implicated in the acute heart valve infection. With the chronic type an entire gamut of germs may be involved, including staph, strep, pneumococcus (usually they are cell wall deficient forms), pseudomonas, Candida, and black mold.

There is a smoldering kind of infection, which, particularly, strikes people with weakened systems. People with a history of a weak heart or weakened heart valves are especially vulnerable. There is another category of high vulnerability: people with weakened adrenal glands. In general it is the thin and slightly weak person who is most vulnerable to this syndrome. This is the syndrome of heart lining and valve infection mentioned previously: the chronic type known medically as subacute endocarditis. This infection is usually caused by bacteria, but, again, a wide range of germs may be involved. If untreated, eventually, this will lead to premature death. Thus, the germs must be eradicated.

The disease most commonly occurs in people over 40, particularly those over 50. Apparently, with time the tissues weaken and become more vulnerable to infection. Diseased gums and teeth are an insidious connection: their strength greatly declines with age, which increases the risks for sepsis. This is also the age, that is between ages 45 to 70, when high blood pressure becomes epidemic. Thus, aging, gum disease, and high blood pressure are closely connected. The weakened or degenerated gums increase the risks for the seeding of infection. If there is heart valve or heart lining infection, there is a high likelihood for the development of high blood pressure.

This condition is more common than is recognized. It is often misdiagnosed, for instance, as a mere heart murmur or mitral valve prolapse or perhaps valvular scarring, for instance, aortic stenosis. In all cases the likely cause is infection: within the heart itself, although this too arises from elsewhere. This is especially if scarring of tissue is discovered. Infection is an enormous stress upon this organ. For optimal health and longevity such an infection must be eradicated. Again, it was Rahimtoola who made it clear that the heart valves are commonly infected, notably by bacteria. The mitral valve is the most commonly affected site, which gives credence to a simple fact: the majority of cases of mitral valve prolapse are probably infective. What's more, those who have undergone valve replacement surgery are likely to have valvular infections, as are a high percentage of those who have had bypass surgery. Another high risk group are surgical patients, who have catheters placed in their veins and, particularly, arteries.

The prolonged use of urinary catheters may also result in heart valve infection. The long-term IV administration of drugs may also lead to heart infection. The drugs themselves weaken the immune system. IV catheters stimulate germ growth. After such catheter use the most commonly found germs in the heart include the tough-to-kill staph, pseudomonas, and candida. Yet, the surgical implantation of any foreign device, particularly shunts and stints, may ultimately lead to heart valve infection. This is also true of various devices which are placed systematically such as artificial joints, metal plates, and spinal rods. The fact is any foreign body breeds infection. Consider this: when there is a mere splinter under the skin, it always becomes inflamed as well as infected. Then, what would reasonably develop with an artificial device planted deep within the tissues?

The fact is any invasion of the body, particularly through major surgeries, readily causes this condition. By far the greatest number of surgeries are performed in America. Here, financial motives play a significant role. This is why in North America sepsis is one of the main causes of death. According to the *Journal of the American Medical Association* as many as 250,000 Americans die yearly of medically induced sepsis, a disease which, previously, was rare. Incredibly, prior to the early 1900s death from sepsis was essentially unknown.

It has already been mentioned how germs from the mouth can infect the heart. Even highly orthodox sources, such as

Rahimtoola, confirm this. He describes research documenting how even mere chewing or grinding of the teeth can spurt germs from the mouth into the bloodstream. The germs may or may not infect the inner tissues, that is the internal organs. What is certain is that after invasive dentistry, even mere teeth cleaning, dozens of different oral microbes can be found in the blood. One study showed, using blood cultures, that within five minutes of a dental procedure large numbers of oral bacteria could be found within the blood. In most instances the immune system will clear them. However, if an individual is compromised or suffering from a weak organ, then infection may set in. Yet, only rarely do the germs directly attack the heart. Rather, they accumulate in clumps of blood tissue, the so-called thrombin clot. Here, in the rich blood-born environment they flourish. The clot essentially becomes a microbial clump, and it becomes sticky. Ultimately, it enters the heart, where it may become lodged, leading to infection. Yet, the clumps also clog arteries, which can block the blood supply. Oxygen starved, the tissues die, and infection sets in. So, it is the combination of congealed or clotted blood plus the germ that creates the infection.

If the blood is naturally thin and extraordinarily healthy, the likelihood of septic infection of the heart, even after invasive therapies, is nil. This demonstrates the need for prevention as well as treatment. The treatment is to destroy both the clots and the infection. The prevention is to keep the blood, as well as gums, relatively germ-free, plus to keep the blood relatively thin. Yet, incredibly, if the infections are eradicated, the blood naturally stays thin. This is because germs, in fact, create stickiness of the blood. They are more dangerous in this regard than even fatty foods. It is to their advantage to create bizarre clumps, so they can cling to them, feed off of them, and hide in them. Then, they can evade the immune system and proceed to infect critical tissues such as the lungs, brain, kidneys, and heart. Here, they hide within the organs and within the organs' cells, evading the immune system and, thus, causing chronic infections. The danger is undeniable. What's more, there is no medical cure. This is why combination therapy using a variety of natural medicines is of such value. Regarding diseases of circulation only nature has the answers. These are stubborn conditions, so a multiplicity of therapies is ideal. As mentioned previously the mainstay of treatment is the edible spice oils. Yet, potent enzymes, which root out the inflammation, are also invaluable. The Infla-eez, which is strictly plant-source, is ideal for this purpose. This is an enzyme concentrate, which is specific for cleansing all blockages from the circulatory system. What's more, potent flavonoids, which inhibit blood clotting and which relax and strengthen the arterial walls, are critical. For this purpose the Resvital powder or capsules is used. High doses may be necessary to rapidly reduce blood pressure. Natural vitamin C is needed, that is to prevent scarring and keep the blood vessels, as well as veins, in as strong a condition as possible.

Natural vitamin C is well absorbed as well as well tolerated. In contrast to synthetic vitamin C, which can cause digestive upset, with the natural type digestive disturbances are unknown. Natural vitamin C is available as Purely-C, which is available both in capsules and liquid form. Regarding the spice oil extracts the OregaBiotic and Oreganol (i. e. the oil of wild oregano) are most critical. The OregaBiotic is, essentially, a spice oil-based antibiotic, with the ability to act as a systemic treatment. This formula is the original garlic, oregano, cumin, and allspice oil concentrate therapy, which is based upon Cornell University research. It is of unequaled power in its ability to kill a broad range of germs. Oil of clove buds plus oils of oregano and cinnamon (OregaDENT) as well as oil of propolis (PropaHeal) are additional potent therapies. Note that the OregaBiotic is ideal for two reasons: it kills germs plus it provides extracts of highly cardioprotective substances such as garlic and wild P73 Oreganol.

All components of the bloodstream are fully connected. Whatever influences a portion of it will influence its entirety. Disease in any region, including the mouth, can affect the remainder of the body. If there is disease in the mouth, this can be readily transferred to the blood and, thus, to the internal organs. In *Infective Endocarditis* the link is made clear, "Strong evidence implicates (dental) procedures as precipitating causes of endocarditis." Notice the use of the word, "cause." Thus, the majority of cases of this life-threatening infection arise from the dentist's chair. Incredibly, if the blood of patients is evaluated after such procedures up to 30% have evidence of major bacterial counts: all arising from the mouth. Thus, the first source to consider for seeding this infection is always the mouth, the gums, and the teeth. A thorough dental history must be performed, with emphasis on the history of pulled teeth, invasive gum surgery, and root canals. The potential chronic seeding of germs from seemingly stable but toxic teeth, such as filled or capped teeth or implants, must also be considered. In some instances there may be need to extract poisoned teeth. Yet, this must be done cautiously, for risk of further seeding the infection and causing, perhaps, a medical crisis. The alternative is to treat the gums and teeth with natural antiseptics as well as to use such antiseptics to cleanse the blood. This will suffice in the majority of cases, yet, in many instances extraction of the suspect teeth is necessary.

The spice oils, such as the Oreganol and OregaDENT, are particularly valuable in the treatment of this condition. This is largely because of their solvent action, which causes these oils to penetrate all tissues. What's more, endocarditis is largely spread through the lymphatic system, and spice oils act aggressively upon this system. The spice oils readily enter the lymphatics, sterilizing them. Thus, the regular use of these oils will largely prevent, as well as reverse, septic diseases. What's more, since spice oils are solvents they help dissolve deposits in the blood. It is these deposits, which are often sticky, which encourage the infection.

By eliminating the sticky deposits in the blood, infections can be cured as well as prevented. Clumpy blood is a major precursor of infection. The wild spice oils halt this process. What's more, there are certain enzymes, which are capable of dissolving clotted material. Notably, Infla-eez, which is an exceedingly potent type of bromelain and papain, aggressively dissolves clots as well as all other sticky arterial matter. The combination of the enzymes plus spice oils routinely cures this condition.

For stubborn conditions propolis may prove invaluable. Propolis has immense healing properties and helps prevent scar tissue formation. It is also a source of bioflavonoids, which help strengthen gum tissue. Oil of propolis (i. e. PropaHeal) is an emulsion of the essential oils, plus wild propolis. Like the oil of oregano it may be applied directly to the gums as well as taken internally.

The heart may also be infected by fungi. These fungi aggressively attack the inner lining of the heart; however, regarding such a deep-seated fungal infection it is difficult to make the diagnosis. It must be presumed based upon history. Invasive medical therapy, as well as invasive dentistry, are the major risk factors for spreading fungal infection. The treatment is the same: the extensive use of wild spice oil extracts. However, it may need to be prolonged: up to six months. Even, a rather rapid improvement should be expected. It was a study at Washington D. C.'s Georgetown University which documented the immense powers of wild spice extracts, particularly the Oreganol P73, in the eradication of fungal infections. Despite the development of systemic infections, that is infection of the blood and internal organs, within 30 days all traces of this germ were eradicated from the tissues. This study, published in *Molecular and Cellular Biochemistry,* is a landmark proving that natural medicines are equal, in fact, superior, to synthetic drugs.

The white cells are capable of killing Candida, however, it is an exhaustive job. Wild oregano extracts greatly aid the white blood cells, by providing their internal workings with antiseptic compounds. In other words, incredibly, the active ingredients in the wild oregano are readily absorbed by the white blood cells, and these substances greatly boost the cells' killing capacity. In contrast, many antibiotics disrupt the function of these cells.

The diagnosis of underlying heart valve or arterial infection is not always easy. It takes an astute, trained physician to do so. Under the nail bed there can be tiny splinter-like lesions, which have a blood-like color. These are known as splinter hemorrhages. Tiny blood blisters on the skin are also common, which are known as petechiae. In the extreme the skin can be hot and tense. There is usually fatigue, with difficulty climbing steps or undergoing exertion. Shortness of breath is an ominous sign. In the acute phase there is fever and often a heart murmur. In the chronic type some 90% of all patients have a murmur. In about one fourth of the cases there is significant joint pain. With a sudden or acute case of this disease, that is the truly life-threatening form, the symptoms include fever, chills, sweats, no appetite, nausea, headache, shortness of breath, difficulty breathing, and chest pain. All these symptoms may not be present. Yet, a combination of the majority of these symptoms is ominous. Untreated, in the majority of the cases death occurs.

Arterial infection: a shocking reality

Doctors, as well as the general public, have always regarded arterial disease as a dietary or toxic issue. The focus has been on the role of diet and, particularly, cholesterol, in the cause of plugged or hardened arteries. Yet, the fact that human arteries are readily infected is undeniable. Virtually any artery can be infected. In some instances, such as in various forms of vasculitis, the entire arterial tree may become inflamed and/or infected. In sepsis, which afflicts some 500,000 Americans yearly, all the arteries are involved.

It makes sense that arteries are infected, especially diseased and stiff ones, such as the arteries of atherosclerosis. The word sclerosis, that is scarring, is revealing. Infection is the main cause of scar formation in the body. Entire diseases once thought to be due to unknown causes, such as aneurysm, vasculitis, stroke, nephritis, and arthritis, are now proving to be infective in origin. The infective nature of aortic aneurysm is well established. The fact is germs readily destroy the arterial walls and may largely cause the condition. Experiments have proven that if the arterial wall is weakened, germs may enter it, causing its destruction. This results in an aneurysm, which is, essentially, a weakening or ballooning of the arterial walls. Once such a lesion forms unless the infection is aggressively destroyed, premature death is likely. Upon the destruction of the infection most aneurysms stabilize, and the risk for sudden death declines dramatically.

Aneurysms may have their origin in infection. Germs are highly destructive. They can readily damage tissue, including the rather tough arterial walls. Once the walls are sufficiently weakened the artery balloons out, and an aneurysm develops. Yet, usually, it begins with infection. This infection often arises from a distant region, settling on the heart valves. The most common culprits are staph and strep, although, increasingly,

Candida is being discovered. As a result of the pumping action of the heart the infection can be seeded to infect virtually any artery, including the arteries in the brain. What's more, the entire arterial tree is well supplied with lymphatic vessels. Conceivably, the germs would migrate from the site of infection, potentially infecting the entire arterial system. Yet, the most likely result is a gradual spread from the site of origin, for instance, from the heart valves to the closely associated aorta.

The body makes every conceivable effort to destroy this infection. Yet, often, it is overwhelmed. What's more, these infections are largely due to drug-resistant germs: freaks of nature. The immune system has a difficult time destroying such germs. Furthermore, these germs are located in difficult-to-reach areas such as the heart valves and inner linings of the arteries. Thus, the body needs help. That help comes from wild spice oils. Such oils are from edible species of plants, so they can be taken with impunity. In other words, without concern they can be taken in large amounts over prolonged periods.

The fact that the arteries are readily infected is indisputable. Remember, dentists are obligated to give antibiotics whenever doing invasive procedures, that is on patients with weak hearts. Yet, such treatment should be routine regardless of the patient's health, as is demonstrated by the following:

CASE HISTORY:

Mr. M., a 50-year-old white male, had no history of heart disease. Then, suddenly, he fell over on his kitchen table, the victim of a heart attack. He was diagnosed with a bizarre condition: the sudden splitting of his heart valve, a condition which could only occur as a consequence of infection. Yet, his doctors never suspected the connection.

I met this couple well after the incident. A thorough history was performed. It was determined that prior to the heart attack Mr. M.

had essentially excellent health, with the exception of his dental system. Recently, some six months before his heart attack he had undergone extensive dental procedures, including root canals. The surgery had not gone well, and he suffered from complications. He began to notice increasing fatigue, and his wife told him, "It's those bad teeth that are bothering you." However, no one knew how truly toxic his reaction was, that is until his heart attack.

There is an excessive focus on the role of diet in heart disease. Compared to the role of infection diet has a minimal impact. True, diet is critical. Surely, the high intake of processed foods damages the circulatory system. However, it is infection, which can cause sudden death. Thus, its role is far more critical than the role of diet. There is an obvious implication: the focus should be on the infectious sites and their appropriate treatment—this is where the therapy must begin. What's more, as a result of successfully eliminating the infectious connection the diet therapy will be more effective.

Infections within the bloodstream, heart, and arteries are highly dangerous. The source of such infections is usually the mouth, that is the gums, teeth, and surrounding bone. Treatment should be aimed at destroying the infections within this region. The Oreganol P73, as well as the OregaDENT, are ideal for this purpose. The fact is the OregaDENT, a combination of edible wild oregano, cinnamon, and clove oils, is specifically formulated for this purpose. This combination offers both antiseptic and anesthetic actions. Plus, it has an excellent taste.

Heart valve infection is far more common than is medically recognized. Nearly one in five Americans suffer from it. This is perhaps a conservative estimate. For instance, up to 90% of Americans suffer from gingivitis, that is infection and inflammation of the gums. In such individuals a certain degree of heart valve and/or arterial infection is assured. What's more, regarding surgical patients as many as half may experience at least a temporary infection of the heart and arteries. Usually, the circumstance are more ominous: the development of a chronic, smoldering infections, which insidiously deplete health, not through acute symptoms but rather through chronic debilitation.

At all costs such infections must be purged from the body, that is if the individual is to experience vital health. It is the spice oils which can effectively achieve such a purge. Since such oils are, in fact, natural foods, they can be taken in large amounts, without concern. There is a word of caution: make sure the spice oils that are consumed are true foods, that is from food grade materials. The North American Herb & Spice Co. wild oregano oil and similar oils are derived from fully edible plants. Beware of imitation formulas, which are extracted from inedible, even toxic, plants. For instance, recent studies have shown that generic sources of oil of oregano are derived from certain herbs, which are not edible. Beware of cheap imitations. Only the P73 oil is safe to take on a daily basis and in large amounts. What's more, the P73 edible spice oil taken as directed is even safe during pregnancy and nursing.

Chapter 3

Chemicals That Kill

The body consists of chemicals. It is truly a chemical soup. It may appear solid, however, it is nearly all fluid. It consists of mainly water, followed by protein, minerals, vitamins, fatty acids, and various trace substances.

It is easy to understand why the old saying, "You are what you eat," is true. A person's chemical soup is based on what he/she eats, drinks, and breathes. Whatever chemicals which are consumed become the basis of human bodies. If these chemicals which are consumed are natural and nourishing, the person will have vital health. His/her resistance will be strong. In contrast, if such chemicals are synthetic and noxious, there will be poor health, unhealthy appearance, and weakened resistance. This is the law of biology as well as biochemistry. There is no other possibility: again, people consist precisely of what they eat as well as breathe and drink. Thus, be wary of what you put in your body. Only you can control this. Only you can determine how you shall live—or die.

The heart and arteries are highly sensitive to toxic chemicals. So are all other organs, particularly the glands. It is the glands, primarily the adrenals and thyroid, which are directly involved with blood pressure regulation. If such glands are poisoned, then the blood pressure mechanism can fail. This may result in high or low blood pressure. What's more, the nervous system is highly sensitive to toxic chemicals. Many chemicals exert their toxicity on the nerves. Many such chemicals are, in fact, fat soluble.

The nerves are a fatty tissue, as is the brain. Thus, fat soluble poisons readily enter them where they exert destructive actions. If nerve and brain tissue is sufficiently disrupted, their ability to conduct impulses is compromised. The toxins fully interfere with nerve and brain cell activities, leading to a wide range of symptoms, including depression, anxiety, panic sensations, apathy, memory loss, and even seizures. The arteries and nerves have their own array of nerves, which may also be damaged. What's more, the glands, particularly the adrenals, are extensively supplied with nerves. This is a highly vulnerable system. Any toxic stress on the nerve cells, if prolonged and significant, could result in high blood pressure. Thus, it is no surprise that the regular ingestion or exposure to toxins in the food, beverages, or environment increases the risks for this condition.

Alcohol: the number one toxin

Regarding the nervous system alcohol is one of the most destructive substances known. Due to its toxic actions on the nerves it damages the senses. It also damages the blood pressure sensors. What's more, it damages all nerve cells, in fact, kills them. The fact is a typical high ball causes the death of nearly a million brain cells. There is only a limited supply of such cells. Thus, heavy alcohol consumption causes permanent brain damage.

There are a number of reasons alcohol causes high blood pressure. One of the major ones is its effects upon the nerve lining. Alcohol denudes, that is strips, this protective lining. This causes the nerves to become hyper-irritable. It is the nervous system, which controls arterial tone. What's more, alcohol is directly toxic to the heart and arteries. Regular intake causes a thickening of both of these organs. Furthermore, this substance poisons the cardiac cells, especially the energy-producing components known as the mitochondria. The fact is alcohol is directly toxic to heart cells. If consumed persistently, ultimately this results in a condition known as balloon degeneration. This is also known as alcoholic cardiomyopathy. Here, the mitochondria, which are intricate biological machines, turn into mere bloated carcasses of their former selves. What's more, with the loss of their protective coating the nerves themselves may be readily infected. Ultimately, they are destroyed. This is known as alcoholic psychosis, rather, Wernicke-Kosakoff's psychosis. It is a condition in which the brain and nerve cells have been permanently destroyed.

Various vitamins and minerals, which are key to maintaining normal blood pressure, are also depleted by this substance. The gradual loss of such critical nutrients, magnesium, potassium, thiamine, pyridoxine, pantothenic acid, and niacin, ultimately results in hypertension. What's more, the alcohol-induced loss of magnesium, thiamine, potassium, selenium, zinc, and niacin directly damages the heart muscle.

When evaluating a male in his mid 40s to 60s with persistently high blood pressure, I always ask a simple question: how much do you drink daily (or weekly)? The fact is alcohol consumption is the primary factor leading to hypertension in this age group. True, hidden infections play a key role, but alcohol is the precipitating agent.

Alcohol weakens the immune system. What's more, it damages the intestinal, as well as stomach, lining. This increases the risk for various infections. It also increases the risk for cancer. Furthermore, this substance, being a cellular poison, also damages the gums. This further places the individual at risk for sepsis and, thus, heart and arterial diseases.

The direct toxicity of alcohol against gum tissues may largely explain the connection. Alcohol causes severe gum recession as well as bone and enamel loss. The weakened mouth is easily infected by a host of germs. Since alcohol is a solvent, whenever it is consumed the germs are readily dispersed into the blood, wreaking havoc and, ultimately, causing arterial and heart disorders. Since it breaks down the gum lining, the germs aggressively penetrate it, causing chronic infection, even cancer.

Just why alcohol so aggressively destroys nerve tissue is unknown. Yet, the basic fact remains: a single drink, that is a highball, causes the destruction of a million brain cells. Wine, while less toxic, also destroys these cells: hundreds of thousands per glass. Beer also readily destroys them. Incredibly, some people drink several glasses of beer or wine daily. Despite this many people regard it as healthy.

For every glass of alcohol which is consumed the brain suffers permanent damage. This is particularly true in individuals of fine frame and low body weight, for instance, petite women. Alcohol, depending upon the type of drink, also exerts enormous toxicity upon the human liver killing anywhere from a few hundred thousand to several million cells per beverage.

The human brain is incapable of withstanding such insults. Ultimately, it fails. What's more, when the nerves are so extensively damaged, their immune system fails. Thus, they become infected. This at least partially explains the high incidence of hypertension, as well as heart disease, in regular drinkers.

It has been clearly shown that herpes infection plays a significant role in the cause of hypertension. Perhaps in the case of alcoholics it plays a role in brain damage as well as arterial disease.

Alcohol is never a 'health food.' Rather, it is always poisonous. The fact is in order to rapidly reverse hypertension its consumption must be avoided. This is because regarding the blood pressure control mechanism alcohol is a fulminant poison.

An average of two alcoholic drinks per day is sufficient to cause a severe case of this disease. Again, a major reason for its devastating effects is its toxicity to the oral membranes. Alcohol destroys the mucous membranes of this region, increasing the risks for a wide range of oral infections. These infections seed germs into the blood, ultimately causing heart and arterial disorders. The greatest factors for causing their spread are invasive procedures, including dental surgery and intubation, as well as alcoholism. Thus, despite a supposed benefit, that is the positive actions of the wine flavonoids, the negative effects of the alcohol far outweigh any benefit. For high blood pressure sufferers alcohol must be strictly avoided. There can be no positive benefit from its consumption.

Alcohol is highly addictive. Even if a person knows it is toxic, he or she may be unable to quit. This is largely due to its destructive actions on the nutrients. People become so deficient in key nutrients that they crave the temporary sensation that alcohol creates. When the nutrients are systematically replenished, the desire for alcohol is eliminated. Thus, alcoholism is a nutritional disease, and, what's more, it must be treated nutritionally.

The diet for alcoholics must be low in starch. The liver requires protein. In fact, in the treatment of liver diseases high protein diets are a mainstay. The high protein diet prevents blood sugar fluctuations, which are the alcoholic's doom. Starches are the raw materials for making alcohol, and, thus, it is no surprise that alcoholics are intolerant to them. Thus, in particular, barley, barley malt, wheat, corn, rye, and potatoes, all of which are used as raw materials for alcohol production, must be prohibited from the diet. This alone will usually lead to a massive improvement. What's more, the intake of refined sugar must be strictly curtailed. Obviously, all alcohol beverages must be eliminated.

Alcoholics thrive on a strict high protein plus vegetable diet. In other words, this is a sugar- and grain-free diet. As a result of such a diet they experience a dramatic reduction in the cravings for alcohol, in fact, this diet helps reverse the condition. Again, in this plan no grains are allowed. This is because eating grains perpetuates the addiction. Again, to successfully treat this disease, there must a dramatic change in the diet plus the intake of the appropriate nutritional supplements. This is thoroughly covered in the book *How to Eat Right and Live Longer,* (same author) with the alcoholism-reversing chapter, "Alcoholism: the Number Three Killer."

Sugar: the arteries' doom

A major factor in heart disease sugar also plays a key role in the cause of hypertension. The connection between sugar and this disease is indisputable. The relationship between gum and tooth decay and high blood pressure, as well as heart disease, has already been described. Sugar destroys the teeth and gums, creating the environment for infections. In this respect it is largely responsible for the dental factor. What's more, it directly damages the heart and arteries. For ideal cardiovascular health the intake of this substance must be strictly avoided.

Price proved that sugar destroys the gums and teeth, while also depleting the bone mass of the jaw. He then proved that such a process leads to a variety of diseases. In other words, the sugar-induced gum and tooth disease is the precursor. For disease to be prevented proper health and nutrition regarding the dental system must be achieved. Sick teeth and gums lead to a sick body. Sugar is the primary culprit in this regard. It is the refined sugar, which is devastating American society. This is the greatest form of terror inflicted upon this population, in other words, the available food causes disease. This terror is knowingly perpetrated upon the general public, purely for profit. The fact is every day refined sugar devastates the lives of countless millions of Westerners.

It was Bunting who proved the devastating effects of sugar on the dental system and, therefore, the rest of the body. Remember, disease largely begins in the mouth: if the mouth breaks down, the rest of the body follows. What Bunting showed was that by merely restricting poisonous substances, the candy and obvious sugar, there was a reduction in dental disease and an improvement in the structure of the teeth.

People are being killed by food. All that is necessary to revive the health of sick, tired, and lazy children, as well as children with behavioral disorders, is to strictly curtail the intake of sugar. Other sweets need not be restricted, for instance, healthy fruit and wild honey. It is the refined sugar that is the poison. What's more, sugar which is laced with toxic chemicals, such as food dyes and sulfites, is far more toxic than sugar alone. Regarding the danger to American children nutritionist Lyda Roberts takes a strong stance:

> ...no single measure would accomplish more to raise the physical standard of American childhood than the marked restriction in the use of sugar. It would be a decided advantage if it were possible to have a zone around school buildings in which the sale of candy could be prohibited.

In the book, *The Vitamins in Health and Disease,* asserts, "If any radical change is to be made in the American diet, it would be well to replace large quantities of sugar...by potatoes." It is important to note here that children love potatoes, which are a rich source of a wide range of nutrients, even vitamin C, while sugar is not only devoid of such nutrients: it destroys them. This is delineated by a letter published in the *JAMA* by Boston's Dr. R. A. Guy, who decades ago made clear the destructive nature of dietary sugar:

> ..the excessive consumption of sugar...is detrimental to the public health...a quarter of the caloric intake in the form of sugar makes a sufficiency of B vitamins almost impossible...The public should be brought to understand that sugar, as such is no necessity, and that the energy can better be derived from foods that carry other essential nutrients.

Refined sugar is highly destructive. Of note there was essentially no diabetes in this country, that is until sugar was introduced. The rise in diabetes is directly correlated with sugar consumption. Consider the Yemeni Jews. Living on yogurt, butter, and meat, diabetes was unknown. After moving to Westernized cities they developed this disease in epidemic proportions. Consider also heart disease as well as hypertension. For instance, the Inuit, living on a high fat and animal food diet, were free of these diseases, that is until they adopted a high sugar Western diet. Refined sugar is the most noxious substance in the diet. Its connection to diabetes and heart disease is beyond doubt. Avoid it at all costs.

Nitrated meats: a key threat

Highly destructive, nitrated meats are well known for their ill effects. When ingested, the nitrates in these meats, which are synthetic chemicals, are converted to dangerous compounds known as nitrosamines. According to Kedar Prasad, Ph.D., nitrosamines are among the most potent carcinogens known. What's more, such compounds are highly toxic to the body's oxygen mechanism, depleting tissue levels of the much-needed nutrients.

Nitrosamines bind to red blood cells, disrupting the flow of oxygen to cells. The lack of oxygen places great stress on the heart, which is forced to pump greater volumes of blood to supply the body's needs. Every dose of nitrated meat places additional stress on this organ. What's more, evidence exists that the regular intake of nitrates in the form of nitrated, that is processed, meats and/or high nitrates in water leads to hardening of the arteries as well as stroke. The fact is nitrates and their highly toxic metabolite, nitrosamine, cause direct toxicity to the arterial wall. Plus, they poison the heart muscle. Ultimately, this may lead to high blood pressure. Furthermore, these chemicals deplete the body of oxygen, which places great stress on the cardiovascular system. Nitrates are particularly dangerous in children, in whom they can precipitate heart disorders. Avoid nitrated foods at all cost. A partial list of such foods includes:

- chipped beef
- bologna
- salami
- Canadian bacon
- ham
- bacon
- hot dogs
- sausage
- bratwurst
- corned beef
- pepperoni
- beef jerky

Pork: the heart's doom

Pork is particularly damaging to the heart. The noxious effects of this substance are demonstrated by the following: an all-you-can-eat contest was offered. Whoever ate a baby roast pig the fastest was the winner. The winner, a 700 pound man, soon became ill. Within a few hours his heart exploded, and he died.

Pork is a harsh meat. It is difficult to digest. It is loaded with microbes. Cooking fails to completely kill its germs. It is well known that pork is one of the most difficult of all meats to digest. There are healthier alternatives. Why consume it, that is when it is so hard on the body?

The great holy books, the Bible, Torah, and Qur'an, prohibit the consumption of pork. The Qur'an is particularly explicit. It proclaims pork as a filthy meat, that is microbially. The modern Bible has been altered; the anti-pork command is no longer specifically written. Yet, it is fully the case that God's messengers, including Jesus Christ and Muhammad, came to reestablish the Mosaic Law, the latter of which prohibits pork. Incredibly, all such messengers established the same dietary code. The fact is this is the code of the great Creator.

I have seen great catastrophes secondary to the consumption of pork: arthritis, heart disease, heart attacks, hypertensive crises, rheumatoid arthritis, lupus, stomach cancer, colon cancer, breast cancer, ovarian cancer, esophageal stricture, pancreatic cancer, esophageal cancer, skin cancer, melanoma, ulcerative colitis, fibromyalgia, vasculitis, and more. Bodies ruined, pork has inflicted great damage upon the human race:

CASE HISTORY:

A new bride, Ms. S. married an Iowa pork farmer. Her new husband insisted on the regular eating of pork, which Ms. S. had never before consumed. Within two years she developed a fulminant case of rheumatoid arthritis. The joint deformities were grotesque, all of which were the consequences of heavy pork consumption. Her body had been overwhelmed by pork parasites, which are not necessarily killed by regular cooking. As a result, she suffers in unmerciful pain.

Certain pork-based germs are encysted, which means they resist heat. When the flesh is ingested, these cysts open up in the human digestive tract, infecting it. Eventually, these pork-derived germs enter the bloodstream, from which they infect the internal organs, including the muscles and the joints. Trichinosis is only one of such germs. For instance, consider the pork whipworm, an encysted parasite which is a primary cause of muscle and joint disease. There are hundreds of such germs within pork. The Bible, Qur'an, and Torah all prohibit it. Why is humankind still eating it? Strictly avoid the consumption of pork.

CASE HISTORY:

A fellow medical student knew that for 'health reasons' I was against the consumption of pork. Being well aware of the damaging effects of this 'food' upon the human body I tried to warn my medical school friends against eating it. One day he approached me, shaking in a clammy sweat. He said, "It got me." He had eaten home-made bratwurst at a barbecue. After developing unmerciful diarrhea, he stated, "it's the most severe sickness I have ever had." Even though the diarrhea finally stopped, he felt incredibly toxic. From his body language it was clear: he knew he had poisoned himself, and, yet, he instinctively knew it was avoidable: simply by following the divine law. Remember, rather than a man-made law it is almighty God who prohibits the consumption of pork.

Pork is hard on the heart as well as the arteries. It directly poisons these organs, largely because of its high microbial load. The microbes readily infect the digestive tract, and from there they enter the bloodstream to infect the internal organs. The heart muscle may also become infected, as is demonstrated by the following:

CASE HISTORY:

A dentist friend of mine invited me for dinner. For his guests he cooked steaks but for himself he insisted upon pork chops. He cooked his chops medium-rare. My colleague, who is always so brave, (she's a woman with the bravery of a legion of men} warned him that pork was hard on the heart and that, surely, cooking it so little would lead to catastrophe. She said to the dentist, "You have the signs of heart disease; you shouldn't eat rare pork." Stubbornly, he quipped, "I don't see any problem—I'm fine." I noticed his fingernails, which bore signs of parasitic infection. I warned him of the same that the pork parasites could attack his heart. About two months thereafter he suffered a massive heart attack and nearly died.

To keep the heart and arteries in good health the consumption of pork must be avoided. This includes pork flesh as well as ham and bacon. Due to its exceptionally high microbial count pork is the poorest meat choice, particularly for those with a history of heart disease and/or hypertension. In particular, in African-Americans it plays a major role in ill health. Untold millions of African Americans have suffered dire disease, as well as premature death, due to the heavy consumption of this meat. Beef is a superior choice, that is organically-raised beef. So is lamb. The latter are herbivores, that is they (should) eat only vegetation. In contrast, pigs are omnivores, which means they eat a variety of food, including animal sources. The fact is any animal which eats other animals is unfit for human consumption. Regarding land creatures only vegetarian animals should be regularly consumed.

The regular consumption of pork is a major risk factor for heart disease. In particular, in African-Americans pork consumption is directly tied to high blood pressure. The combination of pork, refined sugar, and alcohol is deadly. Removing the pork from the diet often results in a noticeable improvement in heart health. The risk for serious heart and arterial disorders will greatly decline. In particular, African-Americans will experience a rather rapid improvement, even with the blood pressure falling to normal. This is particularly the case if the antiseptic purge is followed, that is the intake of the Oreganol and OregaBiotic. For those who fail to improve rapidly, a massive purge is necessary. It may also be necessary to take blood vessel-rebuilding supplements such as the Resvital.

Pork is difficult to digest, plus it contains a vast array of germs, which are not readily destroyed by cooking. These germs are known as encysted parasites, as well as spore-forming bacteria, which may survive normal cooking temperatures. Recall the case history of the man in the all-you-can-eat contest: pork parasites contaminated his blood, causing blood clotting and, therefore, heart attack.

According to Islamic scholars God does not like the odor of humans who eat pork. Yet, who does like the smell of pigs, that is for humans too it is the most offensive odor. Pork is unfit for human consumption. Jesus, Moses, Muhammad, and Abraham avoided, in fact, prohibited, it. Such men are the fathers of much of humankind, Abraham being directly related to the Jews, Christians, and Muslims. Then, why should the individual eat it?

Hydrogenated oils: membrane destroyers

As a general rule fats are safe, that is as long they are pure and natural. In other words, they are safe if they can be readily digested by the body. Hydrogenated, as well as partially hydrogenated, oils are virtually impossible to digest. In fact, such oils are poisonous. When fed to animals, the oils resulted in disease and death. In contrast, butter is readily digested. This makes sense, since it is natural. Despite concerns of its saturated fat content it is harmless, that is if it is truly natural butter. This is the uniqueness of the God-given substances. The famous Harvard nurses study revealed this very finding: women who ate butter instead of margarine, as is popularly thought, having a higher risk for heart disease, in fact, had a reduced incidence, while the margarine eaters had an inordinately high risk.

Man-made oils—particularly margarine and shortening—are impossible to digest. Worse, such oils, which are largely synthetic, damage the body, causing a toxicity that is difficult, in fact, impossible, to repair. Such oils are directly tied to the rising incidence of a variety of diseases, notably high blood pressure, heart disease, stroke, arthritis, and cancer. Why consume them, that is when the evidence points to their harm?

Regarding public health the food industry has a rather sordid history. Foods are produced for mass appeal, never nutritional value. As long as a food has the potential to sell, that is to generate profits, that is the issue. Safety and nutritional needs are rarely if ever considered. Hydrogenated oils were invented in the laboratory without any science to confirm safety. Despite no proof of safety or nutritional value, such oils became incredibly successful commercially. Yet, they poisoned uncountable individuals, causing tissue destruction and vicious diseases: heart disease, hardening of the arteries, high blood pressure, cancer, diabetes, arthritis, lupus, and dozens of others.

The body is incapable of digesting hydrogenated oils. This is a proven fact. What's more, such oils rapidly cause tissue damage, which is largely irreversible. Thus, the only reasonable approach is avoidance. This means the careful reading of labels of all processed foods. It also means that when eating in restaurants a careful effort must be made to assure avoidance. As a rule all fried foods contain hydrogenated oils unless proven otherwise. Before eating such foods ask your server a simple question: What is the food fried in—exactly what type of oil? If the answer is vegetable oil, the food is unfit for human consumption. If the answer is pure olive oil (hopefully extra virgin) or pure butter, then it can be consumed. Ask these questions, otherwise there is a risk of becoming ill. This is because the most common cause of restaurant-related sickness is the consumption of toxic oils. What's more, all deep fried food must be avoided. These are the most toxic foods anyone could consume.

The regular intake of deep fried foods dramatically increases the cancer risks. What's more, the consumption of such foods greatly increases the rate of aging. This is true of both the internal organs and the skin. Huge and/or numerous brown age spots on the skin are common in consumers of deep fried foods. This is largely due to the toxic effects of frying oils on the cell membranes. The fact is such oils aggressively oxidize, that is destroy, these membranes. What's more, they cause a stiffening of the membranes, a kind of intracellular hydrogenation. Thus, as a result of eating these oils the cells, particularly the cell membranes, are directly damaged. The cell membranes protect the body from invasion, by both germs and/or toxins. Once the membranes are destroyed, the cells are left defenseless. Thus, as a result of the regular intake of synthetic fats a variety of degenerative diseases can result, particularly cancer.

At the turn of the century (early 1900s) hydrogenated oils were first popularized. A man had developed an enormous tumor of the throat. He insisted that it was due to deep frying oils. Medical doctors refused to accept it. The man proposed an experiment. In front of a medical school class he insisted that his neck/throat tumor was caused by such oils. The tumor was measured. Then, he ate oil-contaminated food. The tumor was remeasured, and just as he had predicted, it grew significantly. The doctors and medical students were flabbergasted.

Is this anything other than unfathomable? For nearly 100 years it has been known that hydrogenated oils are poisonous. Yet, they continue to be consumed. As a result billions of people are adversely affected. The fact is this is a crime against humanity, a kind of corporate terrorism.

Hydrogenated and partially hydrogenated oils are found in a plethora of processed foods. These oils are extensively used in restaurants, especially in deep fried or batter fried foods. Thus, the human exposure to such fats is vast. This is particularly true of people living in Westernized countries.

Hydrogenated oils are a primary cause of a disease, including the major killers, heart disease and cancer. Research at Harvard University has proven the connection. The regular intake of these oils greatly increases the risks for premature death while in contrast to popular belief the regular use of natural fats, for instance, the fats in beef, whole milk, or butter, failed to increase the risks. In particular, as a result of their regular ingestion in women the risk for breast cancer rises exponentially. The fact is the intake of hydrogenated and partially hydrogenated oils is perhaps the primary risk factor for this disease. Other cancers which may be caused by such oils include colon, pancreatic, stomach, ovarian, and lymphatic cancers. A partial list of the food sources of these oils includes:

crackers	buns
rolls	bread
cereal	fruit pies
breaded foods	batter-fried foods
candy bars	hard chocolates
donuts	sweet rolls
fried chicken	fried fish
cakes	cookies
commercial muffins	waffles and pancakes

creamed frozen vegetables microwave popcorn
commercial granola bars margarine or shortening
French fries hash browns or Tater Tots
pizza (in the crust) toaster pastries
mayonnaise tartar sauce
potato chips, tortilla chips
fried mushrooms, zucchini, hush puppies, etc.
Cheetos, Cheese Nips, corn chips, etc.
fried chicken or other fried foods in restaurants
Cheez Whiz and similar artificial cheese spreads
imitation ice cream, whipping cream, or non-dairy creamers

Score yourself on the above list. If you scored higher than five, that is if you regularly consume five or more of the aforementioned items, you are significantly poisoning your cells with these oils. A score above ten is a warning of severe damage to the heart, immune system, and arteries. A score above 20 warns of impending doom. If the diet is not changed, potentially fatal diseases are imminent. Strictly avoid the consumption of hydrogenated oils. These are among the most poisonous food additives known. Why poison yourself knowingly? Diseases associated with hydrogenated and partially hydrogenated oils include heart disease, hardening of the arteries, hypertension, heart failure, multiple sclerosis, Alzheimer's disease, Parkinson's disease, arthritis, psoriasis, eczema, lupus, scleroderma, and cancer. Hydrogenated and partially hydrogenated oils should be banned from the food supply. The fact is these oils are proven carcinogens.

Refined vegetable oils: oxidizing agents

The refined vegetable oils include the typical salad oils available in the supermarket. Incredibly, they also include supposedly healthy oils such as Canola oil and some types of flaxseed oil. Sesame oil may also be excessively refined, as are peanut, cottonseed, corn, and soy oils. All such oils are harsh on the body. This is because they cause tissue damage through a phenomenon known as oxidation. The oxidative process damages cell membranes, accelerating aging as well as initiating disease. The fact is a number of diseases are directly tied to oxidative damage of the cell walls, including heart disease, hypertension, cancer, arthritis, diabetes, Alzheimer's disease, Parkinson's disease, lupus, pancreatitis, and multiple sclerosis.

The heart and arteries are particularly vulnerable to the toxicity of refined vegetable oils. The problem is these oils oxidize the arterial walls, causing great damage and inflammation. This will ultimately lead to scarring, that is thickening. In this process tumors of the arterial walls, that is atheromas, may form. Ultimately, this may lead to high blood pressure. Especially if heated, refined vegetable oils are among the most potent heart- and artery-destroying agents known. This is because they directly oxidize the arterial walls. Strictly avoid the intake of any such oils.

Aspartame: chemical trigger

This substance is one of the most poisonous synthetic food additives known. It is completely synthetic and contrary to popular belief has no known natural facsimile.The fact is it is a drug made through a chemical process. In the diet it causes a greater degree of toxic reactions than any other chemical additive.

Aspartame is poisonous both to the nervous system and the internal organs. It directly poisons the nervous system, and this may lead to high blood pressure. What's more, this chemical is a major cause of toxic allergic reactions. These reactions may also cause massive inflammation in the arteries, leading to excessive blood clotting. This can predispose the individual to heart and arterial infection as well as stroke. The thickened blood creates pressure against the heart, with the resulting increase in blood pressure. Aspartame is an aggressive neurotoxin. In this regard it can aggravate circulatory disorders. It may also directly poison the heart. The metabolic products of this substance, methanol and formaldehyde, as well as formic acid, are among the most toxic and neurologically active substances known. The symptoms of aspartame poisoning are diverse and include headache (it is a common cause of migraine), sweating, blurry vision, visual loss (which may be permanent), hearing loss, dizziness, numbness, tingling, memory loss, agitation, hyperactive behavior in children, seizures, convulsions, anxiety attacks, abdominal bloating, weight gain, panic attacks, muscle cramps, joint pain, and fatigue. Thus, it is a systemic poison.

Due to its neurotoxicity according to Sargent in her book, *Hard to Swallow: the Truth about Food Additives,* this substance is now being evaluated as a potential cause of chronic fatigue-like syndromes, multiple sclerosis, Alzheimer's disease, post polio syndrome, anxiety neuroses, manic depressive disorders, epilepsy, and Grave's disease. These disorders may be the result of aspartame's metabolites, that is formaldehyde, methanol, and phenylalanine, which are directly toxic to the brain and spinal cord. In fact, nerve cell death has been associated with these substances. In particular, formaldehyde, a significant by-product of aspartame metabolism, causes corrosion of brain and nerve cells. It is also a potent carcinogen. Phenylalanine is a naturally occurring substance, that is an amino acid. However, in excess it too can cause neurological damage.

Obviously, aspartame poisons the nervous system. In high amounts it can even cause nerve cell death. Thus, the regular consumption will eventually cause permanent brain damage.

Heavy metals: circulatory poisons

Heavy metals are among the most toxic substances known. In many instances, heart disease, as well as hypertension, may be due to undiagnosed heavy metal poisoning.

Cadmium and lead are the main culprits. In particular, due to its toxic actions on the kidneys cadmium has been clearly tied to hypertension. Deposits of cadmium have been found in the kidneys of high blood pressure sufferers. What's more, cadmium poisoning may result in kidney disease, including kidney infections and stones.

It is well known that hypertensive crisis is a key symptom of heavy metal poisoning. Lead is a serious factor in hypertension. In hypertensive crises, that is attacks of uncontrollable high blood pressure, lead is a key cause. Cadmium also directly poisons the heart and arteries, resulting in severe scarring and inflammation. Accumulations of either of these heavy metals in the kidneys is directly related to the cause of high blood pressure.

Heavy metals can be purged from the body. This can be done without drugs. Certain herbal remedies are effective at purging them. The GreensFlush system, the wild greens formula and the wild berries formula, is one such remedy. These help aggressively purge from the liver toxic residues. The greens cause the liver to dump toxins, including heavy metals, solvents, herbicides, and pesticides. Then, these toxins are excreted in the stool. This is the ideal and, in fact, safest means to eliminate heavy metals. This is not the same as wheat grass or similar green drinks. This is an extract of unprocessed wild herbal greens—wild dandelion, burdock, nettle, chickweed, and more. It is effective, even in mercury poisoning.

CASE HISTORY:

J. J. is a five-year-old white male with a history of autism. Examination indicates that this happened post-vaccination. There was a suspicion that heavy metal poisoning was involved. Hair analysis determined unusually high mercury levels. The latter could have been derived from the vaccinations, which contain the mercury-laced 'preservative' thimerasol. In addition, the child suffered from unrelenting diarrhea, which was, apparently, a side effect of a mercury-chelating drug. The wild greens flush (that is the GreensFlush) was started, one dropperful twice daily. Within two days his bowels were normalized. In fact, his mother noted that as a result of the greens he had the first truly normal bowel movement in several years. Then, a virtual miracle occurred. J. J., who was fully dysfunctional and incapable of normal activity, completed a full 50 minutes on a treadmill. He felt so strong that he went out to play in the park for a full hour, activities which were unthinkable only days before. The greens gave J. J. seemingly unlimited energy, for the first time since his vaccination injury.

The wild berries drops are also effective. This is because they contain a wide range of organic acids and flavonoids, with natural metal chelating powers. These flavonoids help bind heavy metals, removing them through the urine. What's more, the wild berries extract helps activate kidney cells, improving the flow of urine. This action is ideal for individuals suffering from sluggish kidneys, a common consequence of heavy metal poisoning. To order GreensFlush call 1-800-243-5242.

Heavy metals can also be removed through a special patch designed specifically to extract poisons. A Japanese invention, this patch contains certain substances, including a special kind of Oriental wood vinegar plus ionically charged minerals. This patch pulls toxins through the lymphatics. Known as Kinotakara this is the only researched and tested heavy metal patch available. It is highly effective, particularly for mercury extraction. The residue of the heavy metals can actually be seen on the patch. The Kinotakara patches are available only via mail order. Do not accept cheap imitations. There are many oriental imitations, many of which have proven dangerous. To order Kinotakara call 1-800-243-5242.

Cigarette smoke: systemic poison

The toxic effects of cigarette smoke on the heart and arteries is extreme. Smoke poisons the circulatory system. Smoking directly damages the arteries, as well as heart muscle, precipitating disease. The fact is cigarette smoking is a major cause of premature death due to heart attacks, heart failure, and stroke.

Cigarette smoke destroys the arteries, again, through oxidation. What's more, it causes heavy metal poisoning. Such metals are contaminants in the tobacco. Pesticides and herbicides are also volatilized and absorbed, which are also major contaminants. Thus, tobacco is a systemic poison, which destroys virtually all organs of the body.

If you are a smoker and you expect to have good health and a decent, long life, you must quit immediately. Why ruin yourself with your own two hands? Cigarette smokers are victims of an industry that seeks to manipulate human beings for its own profit. Why buy into it?

In order to heal the body cigarette smoking must be halted. Once the smoking is eliminated the hypertension can be reversed. So can the majority of heart defects, although it will take time to detoxify the residues. Here, the radical change in the diet and nutritional supplements will cleanse the tissues of toxic residues.

Cigarette smoke destroys the body in another way: nutrient depletion. In particular, it destroys vitamin C. A mere cigarette destroys as much vitamin C as is in a small orange. A pack destroys more vitamin C than can possibly be eaten in a day. Why tempt life? Vitamin C is crucial for the workings of the circulatory system, in fact, all systems. It is particularly valuable for the maintenance of arterial health. The arterial walls require it to prevent scar formation and to keep their walls elastic. For heavy smokers there is no means to consume in the diet sufficient vitamin C to neutralize the damage. Smoke destroys the naturally occurring vitamin C in the body. Taking synthetic vitamin C while smoking fails to protect the arteries from the smoke-induced damage. In order to heal the arteries smoking must be halted. To neutralize the damage it is necessary to consume antioxidant-rich spice extracts, such as the Oreganol, Juice of Oregano, and OregaBiotic. Also, consume natural vitamin C, that is Purely-C, as well as crude red sour grape, that is the Resvital. The latter helps regenerate damaged arterial walls.

To reverse the damage from smoking Purely-C should be consumed in large quantities, for instance, three capsules twice daily. Incredibly, a single capsule contains 120% of the RDA of *naturally occurring vitamin C.* The contents include camu camu berries, acerola cherry, *Rhus coriaria,* and rose hips. There is not a single molecule of synthetic vitamin C in this formula. What's more, synthetic vitamin C is largely made from genetically engineered corn. In susceptible individuals this may lead to toxic reactions. The fact is genetically engineered foods, as well as the substances derived from them, are unfit for human consumption.

The Oreganol is also invaluable. It has a specific action for combating stroke-induced damage. It may even help in reversing the addiction itself. This is because a few drops of Oreganol taken under the tongue halts the cravings for tobacco. If done at the moment of every craving, it may halt all desire.

To reverse this there is also the need for adrenal support. This is because tobacco poisons these glands. Thus, a sublingual form of royal jelly, such as the Royal Oil, will greatly aid in reversing the addiction.

Cortisone: doomsday medicine

Regarding the heart and arteries cortisone is no medicine. Rather, it is a deliberate poison. The toxic effects of this substance on the circulatory system are well known. Cortisone causes fluid retention, and this is particularly true of Prednisone. It is a primary cause of high blood pressure as well as fluid retention and obesity. The fact is the heavy use of Prednisone causes its own kind of obesity: a truncal type, where the weight is centered heavily in the abdomen. This is known as Cushing's Syndrome. The syndrome causes a great deal of deformity, both in fat distribution as well as bone structure. Cortisone rapidly causes mineral loss from the bones, leading to a kind of buffalo-hump appearance. The individual also develops weight gain due to sodium retention. This leads to a distortion of the individual's appearance: bloated or pendulous abdomen is common.

The Prednisone-induced weight-gain is extremely difficult to reverse. Thus, again, the side effects are more severe than the disease. Strictly avoid the intake of Prednisone. If currently taking it, have your doctor help you wean off this drug. A supplement which helps in the weaning process is Royal Power. For purposes of weaning take a few capsules every few hours, that is until the drug is eliminated. Continue taking the Royal Power for a few months after weaning, perhaps permanently.

Royal Power is entirely safe. It is a concentrate of the naturally occurring hormones synthesized by bees, that is the royal jelly that is fed to the queen. Other than allergic reactions to bees there is no possible danger in it, rather, only benefits. It helps rebuild the glands which are damaged by the Prednisone/cortisone.

There is another reason cortisone is a killer. It destroys the connective tissue, potentially damaging all organs in the body. The fact is the inner linings of the heart and arteries, including the heart valves, are largely connective tissue. Cortisone weakens these tissues, greatly increasing their vulnerability to infection. The cortisone-weakened tissues are readily attacked by a host of germs, including viruses, bacteria, fungi, and even parasites. Cortisone also damages the white blood cells, as well as the lymph glands, blocking their ability to mount an infection-killing response. This is why individuals who regularly use this drug, even those who regularly use it topically, have an exceptionally high incidence of heart, heart valve, and arterial infection. Furthermore, this drug directly damages the heart valve, leading to inadequate heart function. Plus, it causes its own disease: swollen or enlarged heart syndrome, that is cortisone- and Prednisone-induced cardiomyopathy. Such drugs are also a primary cause of high blood pressure, but, again, one of the reasons is the fact that infections of the circulatory tract are a common consequence of cortisone/Prednisone therapy.

There is yet another debacle: cortisone- or Prednisone-induced vitamin C deficiency. The regular use of these drugs leads to a vast vitamin C deficiency. Unless the vitamin is vigorously replaced great damage occurs. There develops wholesale destruction of the connective tissue, particularly the tissues found in the arterial walls and heart. Thus, it is no surprise that various forms of heart and arterial disease are virtual automatic consequences of these drugs. Vitamin C should be replaced only through natural sources, for instance, fruits and vegetables, as well as natural vitamin C supplements such as Purely-C and Resvital.

Obesity: an ominous threat

In the Western world obesity is a fulminant epidemic. Most people regard it as a disease of overeating. Few people realize it is largely a toxic syndrome. The fact is obesity is a type of chemical or physiological poisoning. Fat cells are deposited to absorb toxins. The intake of noxious chemicals and refined foods has reached an all-time high. It appears that this toxicity and obesity are related. Toxins accumulate in fat tissue. This leads to inflammation and, therefore, swelling. Thus, the toxins directly contribute to weight gain. Without them, obesity would be rare.

This is surely a dramatic theory, however, it is an accurate one. Test this on yourself. Follow the cleansing protocol in Appendix A. Do nothing else, that is except reduce the intake of toxic foods. Then, experience relatively effortless weight loss.

The deposition of fat is a consequence of toxicity, whether physical, emotional, or chemical. Fat cells are laid down as a form of protection. In other words, one of the main causes of the deposition of fat is the ingestion of toxic substances. If the toxins are restricted and only healthy foods are consumed, weight loss will occur. What's more, if the toxins are aggressively purged from the body, weight loss will be rapid and relatively effortless.

Obese people are at a high risk for hypertension. Obesity places great pressure on the heart and arteries. A mere five pounds of excess weight is sufficient to significantly reduce life span. This is due to the extra work the heart must perform. The body must build numerous additional miles of blood vessels to service the fat, incredibly, nearly a mile of additional vessels for every five pounds of extra weight. The heart must service these extra blood vessels. This demonstrates that even a modest degree of overweight has serious consequences.

Infection is another major cause of obesity. Here, fungal organisms are largely the culprits. The fungi feed on sugars, creating toxins. These toxins lead to bloating, water retention, and, therefore, weight gain.

Fat cells are living tissues; they must be serviced with flowing blood. Losing these excess pounds greatly decreases the pressure on the heart, increasing longevity. Thus, naturally thin people live considerably longer than the obese. Regarding this naturally thin people make up the greater percentage of centenarians. The fact is it is rare to find obese centenarians. Dieting is partially the answer. However, it must be a total nutritional plan aimed at rebuilding body function. It is a plan to nourish the body: weight loss is a side effect. For information on how to nourish the body, while losing weight, see the book, *How to Eat Right and Live Longer* (Knowledge House, Dr. Cass Ingram).

The weight must come off, if for no other reason other than the immense strain it places on the heart. Weight loss need not be difficult. There are natural ways to achieve it. The diet in the aforementioned book, with its special section, Two Weeks of Eating Right, is invaluable. The food is luscious and filling. Plus, certain nutritional supplements speed weight loss. The key to this process is blood sugar regulation, which will reduce any temptations. The fact is if the blood sugar mechanism can be bolstered staying firmly to the diet is easy. What's more, there is a need to balance the hormone system. This is also done through the appropriate nutritional supplements. Key nutritional supplements for losing weight include the thyroid-balancing supplement, Thyroset, as well as the adrenal balancing supplement, Royal Power. For blood sugar regulation Oregulin, which is made from multiple spices, is ideal. It helps eliminate the so-called Syndrome X, which is due to excess or abnormal insulin production.

Oregulin: insulin regulator

As long as the insulin response is in disarray weight loss is virtually impossible. Oregulin eliminates this by modulating a normal insulin response. Incredibly, studies show that Oregulin reduces blood sugar by some 40%, while stabilizing insulin activity. The powers of this spice extract complex are demonstrated by the following testimonial:

CASE HISTORY:

G. B. is a 60-year-old woman who suffers from Type 2 diabetes. Her blood sugar has ranged consistently between 185 and 200 and is resistant to medication. She saw an ad for Oregulin but hesitated to buy it, concerned that it was merely promotion. Yet, then, in desperation she tried it. Quickly, her blood sugar normalized, averaging about 125. This is a 40% drop. In her own words she wrote, essentially, "Thank you for creating a product that works. It has given me hope—you've given me confidence—because it truly works." Thus, in humans the same results are being achieved as in the animal studies.

Yet, even if the blood sugar isn't high, even if it is low, Oregulin is curative. This is because in low doses, such as a capsule twice daily, it is highly effective regenerating the pancreas and, therefore, re-balancing the insulin mechanism. This is largely due to its effects on cellular enzyme systems. Oregulin causes a dramatic increase in cellular production of glutathione-S-transferase, a key enzyme for the synthesis of insulin. Thus, it is effective in both high and low blood sugar. In high doses, such as two or three capsules with each meal, it is an effective fat burner. It does so by stabilizing the insulin mechanism and, therefore, preventing excessive fat deposition. Plus, Oregulin contains certain pungent spices, which speed fat burning.

Depending upon the body size or total weight up to four capsules may be taken three times daily, that is with each meal. There is one warning: Oregulin may increase the desire for food—healthy food. The fact is it reduces any desire for harmful, that is fattening, food. Yet, ultimately, by regulating blood sugar it reduces the desire for food, and with its regular intake the need or desire for snacks is virtually eliminated. In general it is an appetite suppressant. Two Oregulin taken with breakfast seemingly eliminates the desire for mid-morning snacks, even lunch. It is the ideal supplement for eliminating sugar cravings and hunger pangs.

Oregulin can help balance the hormone system, especially the adrenal glands. These glands are weakened by stress, high intake of carbohydrates, and a low intake of salt. They are also weakened by chronic or sudden infection. When they are weakened, the body's ability to regulate blood sugar is compromised. When such an individual eats sugar or carbohydrates, even relatively healthy ones, such as whole grains, brown rice, or fruit, the body reacts by secreting excessive hormones. Thus, the carbohydrates/sugars are deposited as fats. Oregulin corrects this. The carbohydrates are combusted as fuel, and fat deposition is halted.

What's more, refined sugar, as well as starchy carbohydrates, such as white flour, white rice, potatoes, and corn, place a certain amount of stress on the adrenal glands. This is because the adrenal glands are responsible for processing carbohydrates and, particularly, handling any drops in blood sugar secondary to the carbohydrate load. When a person eats sugar and/or starch, within a few hours the blood sugar drops. Insulin processes the initial load of sugar: but as it continues to be digested and absorbed, the adrenal glands handle the remaining burden.

It is these glands which are responsible for preventing the blood sugar from suddenly collapsing. What's more, under the stress of a high intake of refined carbohydrates in most instances, they become weakened that is unless there is protection. Oregulin offers this protection. It keeps the blood sugar level from suddenly falling, greatly reducing adrenal strain. This prevents the excessive secretion of cortisone, and it is the latter which causes weight gain. The Oregulin eliminates the cortisone stress response. This is why it is so effective in causing weight loss. What's more, it reduces the need for insulin. It is well known that an excess of insulin causes fat deposition.

Oregulin helps rapidly balance blood sugar. A study published in *Diabetes, Obesity, and Metabolism,* 2004, determined that it safely lowers blood sugar in diabetic animals as much as 40%. This was achieved while significantly reducing blood pressure. Yet, similar results can be seen in humans. The blood pressure is a marker of insulin resistance, the so-called Syndrome X. Thus, Oregulin helps normalize the entire insulin metabolism, effectively reversing blood sugar disorders as well as diabetes.

Obese individuals, who have a hypersensitive insulin response or who suffer from exhausted adrenal glands, are at a high risk for developing hypertension. Any obese individual who also has hypertension is at a high risk for premature death. Through following the diet in *How to Eat Right and Live Longer* and by taking the aforementioned nutritional/herbal supplements this health catastrophe can be avoided. Oregulin regulates insulin. What's more, by regulating this hormone it causes the burning of fat. This is critical for the success of any long-term weight loss plan.

Those extra pounds truly harm their bearers. The pressure placed on the heart by a mere five or ten excess pounds is significant. Imagine the strain from twenty or more pounds—in the fifty pound-plus category it is catastrophic. Every effort must be made to shed the extra weight. Yet, people need aids, that is metabolic support, which naturally speed the burning of fat. Oregulin is precisely that aid.

Cell cleansing: the power of wild greens

While the fat must be burned and the insulin regulated the toxins must also be removed. This is accomplished through the GreensFlush drops. There are two forms: the wild greens and berries. The regular intake of these drops will purge the toxins out of the body, so that the tissues can heal. This will decrease the deposition of fat and, in fact, help the body liberate and burn it. Thus, a required part of any weight loss protocol is detoxification, and the wild green drops are safe, highly active, and effective. This is truly from wild material from the distant north of Canada and, thus, it is relatively free from toxins. Only such remote wild material can be relied upon as a purge.

For moderate obesity take two droppersful of the GreensFlush, that is of each type of drops, twice daily. For severe cases take four droppersful twice daily. For extreme cases take four droppersful three to four times daily. There is a warning: toxic sludge will be dispelled from the body. Until such sludge escapes there may be a sensation of tiredness or toxicity. Incredibly, this can be alleviated by increasing the dose. The wild greens drops are highly aggressive in the removal of a wide range of toxins, including solvent residues, pesticides, herbicides, fungicides, toxic household chemicals, drug residues, and even heavy metals. Such drops greatly activate the liver's ability to purge the body of toxins. This is why they are invaluable for the obese individual. The fact is obesity is largely a disease of the liver. If the function of this organ can be dramatically improved, there can be no such disease. For ideal results take the raw wild GreensFlush with the spice oil formula, LivaClenz.

The GreensFlush system is a requirement of any serious weight loss program. These drops can only be ordered from finer health food stores or via mail order, 1-800-243-5242. Also, as a fat-burning supplement, as well as a means to regulate insulin, the Oregulin must be taken. What's more, the wild oregano aids in fat burning. This is true particularly of the water soluble form, the Juice of Oregano. This 'juice' also regulates appetite. Juice of Oregano may be purchased in finer health food stores.

Drugs: cures or killers?

Originally, modern medicine was virtually based upon the treatment of blood pressure. Since the late 1940s trillions of dollars of anti-hypertensive drugs have been sold. Thus, the market for this disease alone fully established the pharmaceutical houses as the financial leaders, that is in the health care process. Yet, despite the trillions of dollars spent there was no benefit to the population. In other words, no cure has been discovered. Plus, uncountable individuals suffered additional disorders as a result of the drugs, including serious conditions such as congestive heart failure, heart rhythm disturbances, diabetes, and even stroke as well as heart disease itself. What's more, in men impotence is virtually an inevitable consequence of the regular use of such drugs. Thus, as a result of drug therapy the quality, as well as quantity, of life suffers.

An old edition of a medical magazine, the journal *Circulation*, May 1956, is revealing. In it virtually every ad relates to high blood pressure. It is as if the entire medical system is based upon this single disease. On the inside cover there is an advertisement for a diuretic drug for congestive heart failure and kidney disorders, although due to its high fatality rate it is no longer used.

The claim is that in order to reverse the disease sodium and water must be purged from the body, that is volume depletion. This is surely no cure. At the bottom of this page is an advertisement for a salt substitute made from synthetic potassium and ammonium. The next page shows a physician holding a blood pressure device, faced by a stocky man—the classic hypertensive patient. It is an advertisement for the drug, Apresoline, which, again, forces fluid out of the body. Drugs are repeatedly advertised, proving that this is to a large degree a manufactured disease. Incredibly, it is difficult to turn the pages, that is without discovering an ad for high blood pressure drugs. High blood pressure is merely a symptom. The disease originates elsewhere, usually from some form of systemic toxicity or infection. If the cause can be found and the cure prescribed, the symptoms will be resolved: permanently. What would happen if high blood pressure was never discovered or treated: if there were no device to measure and diagnose it? Due to the reduction in medications people would probably live longer. This is because invasive treatment, as well as drug therapy, fails to, overall, save lives. This is clearly shown by the results of the 1970s era physician strike in New York City. In a mere six months there was a significant increase in life span, which is further proof of the dangers of modern medicine.

Anti-hypertensive drugs are responsible for a significant number of premature deaths. The elimination of the use of these drugs would save uncountable lives. So, if they are killers, how can they be considered as lifesaving? In other words, with high blood pressure the treatment is more dangerous than the disease. A great fraud has been perpetrated against the people, while, incredibly, they are largely unaware of it.

The toxic effects of drugs: nutrient depletion

It is well known that anti-hypertensive drugs deplete nutrients. Many of these drugs are diuretics, which means they cause water loss. Water cannot be lost by itself: nutrients follow. Incredibly, many of the nutrients depleted by such drugs are the very ones which help maintain normal blood pressure: thiamine, vitamin B_6, potassium, calcium, and magnesium. Even sodium and chloride, which are aggressively depleted by certain drugs, are needed for keeping the blood pressure normal.

I have evaluated hundreds of people, who are on high blood pressure drugs. All such people have severe mineral deficiencies. The deficiencies are directly due to the drugs. One way the degree of the deficiency can be determined is by looking at the nails. Individuals who have been on anti-hypertensive drugs for prolonged periods have heavy ridging of the nails, a clear sign of systemic mineral deficiency. The face is also revealing. Enlarged facial pores are often evident, a sign of magnesium as well as B_6 deficiency. If the eyes are bloodshot and there are tiny bright red blood vessel-like lesions around the nose, on the cheeks, or on the tip or bridge of the nose, there is a severe riboflavin deficiency. As a result of the daily intake of such drugs, all the key nutrients needed to control blood pressure: thiamine, niacin, riboflavin, vitamin B_6, magnesium, calcium, potassium, sodium, and chlorides, are readily destroyed and these nutrients must be replaced. For ideal blood pressure control to be maintained there must be a steady supply of such minerals and vitamins.

Yet, it is not merely about control. It is about getting to the cause of this condition. Surely, the nutrients must be replaced. Yet, even this will fail to fully correct the problem. The deeper causes must be reversed. This is accomplished through spice oil therapy, which destroys both the infections and the inflammation, which is responsible for this condition. Only edible spice oils made from naturally occurring wild material must be used. This can be achieved through the intake of the OregaBiotic multiple spice capsules as well as the well known oil of wild oregano (i. e. P73 Oreganol).

Fear is a plague. In fact, fear creates disease. Trust cures it. Thus, there is an advantage in placing trust in the powers of nature or, rather, in the powers of almighty God. There are benefits people can gain from such an approach. The fact is people who live in America already do this. This is because people trust in the Western system, that is in capitalism. Trust in God is supposedly the basis of this system; this is the motto on the dollar bill. Yet, to trust in the truly natural, that is the divinely made, the provisions, which are given to humankind, this is the answer for innumerable diseases.

Spices, particularly their potent oil extracts, are one such provision. So are natural or organic foods. So are raw honey and vinegar. It was almighty God who made such substances. How else could they have occurred? There is every reason to trust in their powers. Thus, people can trust freely in such medicines. This is because natural medicines, which are completely unprocessed and preserved in their naturally powerful state, can never do harm. The fact is the only significant side effects are unforeseen health benefits, like a longer more vital life, greater energy, and improved digestion. In contrast, such side effects never occur with synthetic drugs, which only cause misery and, certainly, in the case of high blood pressure drugs, premature death. It is the North American Herb & Spice company, which specializes in such truly natural unprocessed substances.

Yet, again, a key issue is the fact that natural substances boost the body's functions, while drugs interfere with it. This is certainly true of the interaction of drugs with nutrients. A partial list of drugs which destroy nutrients includes:

Drug	Nutrient destroyed/depleted
aspirin	vitamin C, bioflavonoids, vitamin B_{12}, thiamine, iron, magnesium, vitamin E
antibiotics	vitamin C, vitamin B_{12}, folic acid, thiamine, riboflavin, niacin, zinc, vitamin K, calcium, vitamin A
cortisone/Prednisone	vitamin C, vitamin B_{12}, folic acid, thiamine, riboflavin, vitamin A, vitamin D, zinc
antiinflammatory drugs	vitamin C, vitamin B_{12}, iron, copper,

folic acid, thiamine, vitamin A, vitamin K, vitamin D, zinc

coumadin   vitamin C, vitamin E, vitamin K, vitamin A

antacids   thiamine, pyridoxine, vitamin B_{12}, folic acid, vitamin A, calcium, iron, magnesium, copper

acid-suppressing drugs   vitamin B_{12}, folic acid, thiamine, iron, calcium, magnesium, vitamin B_6, pyridoxine, niacin

cholesterol-lowering   vitamin B_{12}, vitamin A, vitamin D, vitamin E, vitamin K, essential fatty acids, coenzyme Q-10

diuretics   thiamine, pyridoxine, calcium, magnesium, potassium, zinc, riboflavin, sodium, chloride

birth control pills   vitamin E, thiamine, niacin, pyridoxine, folic acid, vitamin B_{12}, vitamin D, vitamin K, zinc

chemotherapy   all vitamins, particularly vitamins C, A, B's and E; selenium, zinc, magnesium, coenzyme Q-10, superoxide dismutase, taurine, folic acid, vitamin C, essential fatty acids, pantothenic acid, beta carotene,

caffeine	thiamine, pyridoxine, niacin, folic acid, calcium, potassium, zinc, magnesium, chromium
mineral oil	vitamins A through K, coenzyme Q-10, essential fatty acids
laxatives	magnesium, sodium, chloride, potassium, zinc
tobacco	selenium, zinc, vitamin C, vitamin A, vitamin E, folic acid, niacin, coenzyme Q-10, vitamin B_{12}
mood-altering (Prozac, Xanax, etc.)	thiamine, pyridoxine, folic acid, vitamin B_{12}, choline, inositol, vitamin C, selenium, magnesium, glutathione

Here is the key. Rather than depleting or destroying them food, herbs, and wild medicines provide nutrients. That is the essential difference between natural medicines and synthetic drugs. The fact is the divinely made substances enhance the body, *boosting* the levels of nutrients. In contrast, synthetic, that is man-made substances, particularly drugs, *detract* from it, while destroying nutrients.

Antibiotics: insidious factors?

The role of antibiotics in the cause of high blood pressure has never before been discussed. It was Lida Mattman, Ph.D., the top scientist in the field of mutated germs, who made the connection. Although she failed to mention it as such her work proves that antibiotics play a direct role in the cause of cardiovascular diseases. This is due to the creation of mutated germs, known medically as cell wall deficients. They are called cell wall deficients, because they have mutated to a form devoid of cell walls. This is largely to evade the effects of antibiotics, which act upon the cell walls. By converting into a cell wall deficient form, they neutralize the antibiotics. In other words, the cell walls are the means by which the immune system recognizes germs. Without these walls, the germs operate in a stealth mode. Such forms neutralize the immune system's attempts to kill them, since this system is dependent upon the cell wall in order to kill bacteria. This mutation, that is this lack of a cell wall, is the germ's adaptation to survive.

The cell wall deficients are to a degree a natural form; antibiotics merely accelerate their growth. These microbes are also known as L-forms, so named for the Lister Institute, where they were first discovered. Their existence has been known since the mid-1800s. However, they have become epidemic as a source of infection only more recently: since the dawn of the antibiotic era.

Mattman has documented how the arteries, as well as blood clots, are contaminated with such germs. These germs secrete potent substances, which cause blood clotting, while damaging the arterial walls. This arterial wall damage, combined with the blood clotting, that is the increased stickiness of the blood, leads to high blood pressure. Yet, it can also result in more ominous consequences: stroke, heart attacks, and sudden death.

The L-forms are active in the bloodstream, and they are found in virtually all Westerners. They are particularly prolific in recipients of mega-antibiotic therapy. Anyone who has taken antibiotics repeatedly is contaminated with such forms. This is also true of those who have taken significant doses of antifungal antibiotics such as Nystatin and Diflucan. Such individuals are contaminated with fungal cell wall deficient forms. The degree of contamination is directly due to the amount of antibiotics taken. Antibiotics fail to kill these forms. Only natural antiseptics can do so. Antibiotics can precipitate various forms of heart disease. Such drugs create a highly destructive reaction. This is the actual creation of bizarre and mutant germs, which readily evade the immune system and, therefore, grow in vast numbers. From a microbiological point of view, such germs may grow into enormous sizes; thus, they cause mechanical damage, that is they obstruct the circulation. Numerous investigators have proven that bizarre germs invade or perhaps create clots, which can become lodged in the heart and/or coronary arteries, leading to disastrous consequences. What's more, antibiotics, being largely poisons derived from fungi, may cause toxic reactions. People who are sensitive to mold and fungus may suffer violent reactions to such drugs. This may lead to water retention, inflammation, and, therefore, hypertension. People who are on the plan in this book must avoid the intake of antibiotics. Antiseptic oils are, in fact, more effective than antibiotics without the risk of side effects.

Food additives: chemicals that kill

The human body is a constructed one by the cells and organs within it. These cells depend upon what a person eats and drinks, truly each person is made up of what he or she consumes.

Chemicals, that is synthetic food additives, are not meant for nutrition; the body never benefits from them. Rather, they are used by the food processors to supposedly enhance the attractiveness of the foods. The fact is all they can enhance is the further destruction of the body. Foods contain chemicals, but these are the ones needed by the body which the body readily recognizes: amino acids, fatty acids, coenzymes, vitamins, and minerals. A person can build a healthy body with these. In contrast, synthetic chemicals interfere with body building. They disrupt the process, leading to a weakening of cells and organs. A person should guard what he/she consumes. If a food contains a man-made substance, then the food should be avoided.

There is evidence that hypertension could in part be an allergic disease: to toxic chemicals in the food. What's more, arterial damage, as well as general organ damage, has been tied to their intake. It was the British researcher, Dr. Franklin Bicknell, in his monograph, *Chemicals in Food*, who made it clear that noxious additives in food, while not always causing sudden death, by "gnawing away at the body" lead to "goiter, coronary thrombosis, disseminated sclerosis (i.e. multiple sclerosis), cancer, etc." After reviewing the scientific literature Bicknell makes the following recommendations:

• Chemical food dyes serve no nutritional purpose. They should be avoided. Candies, cakes, icings, ices, canned peas, and similar foods, which contain artificial colors should not be eaten. These synthetic dyes are cancer-causing, what's more, they may cause brain damage.

• No artificial emulsifiers should be consumed; in fact, they should never be added to the food; this includes polysorbate 80, ethylene glycol, and propylene glycol—all such chemicals are cancer-causing. What's more, toxicity tests show that the ingestion of such chemicals causes damage to the kidneys, colon, and bladder, even causing bladder stones.

• Never eat commercial or white bread; never eat any white flour-based food, including buns, rolls, and pasta. Such food is unfit for human consumption, in fact, dangerous. This is largely due to the bleaching process, through the use of chlorine gas. The chlorine creates highly toxic compounds, which damage the body. The arteries take the brunt of the damage, as these chemicals become volatilized in the bloodstream. Incredibly, despite processing, flour contains vitamin E prior to chlorination, but this harsh process completely destroys it. Thus, white flour is vitamin E-free; the most important heart and artery-protective compound has been destroyed. Residues of chlorine remain— essentially the same compound as bleach—and this creates toxic derivatives, including bizarre chlorinated fatty acids. Such derivatives readily cause tissue damage, even cancer. A type of highly toxic methionine is created, which greatly interferes with cardiac function. What's more, as has been demonstrated by Price, chlorine itself has been proven to cause circulatory diseases. Ominously, Bicknell claims that the food processors, in their manufacturing of white flour, have made a food, which is "as insidiously corrupting to the body as a food can well be." Plus, he makes a compelling recommendation that "Mothers must make their family's bread, etc., from untreated stone ground flour from small mills."

• Margarine of any type should not be eaten. Such fats are usually contaminated with pesticides, which were used in the growing of the seed, from which the oils were derived. What's more, margarine directly antagonizes one of the body's most key nutrients: essential fatty acids. A margarine-induced essential fatty acid deficiency increases the risks for hardening of the arteries, skin diseases, and cancer. In Britain the rising incidence of arterial diseases is not correlated with butter intake but, rather, with the intake of margarine. In contrast, during World War II the Norwegians experienced a decline in heart disease: their margarine factories had been destroyed by the Germans. What's more, margarine, that is hydrogenated oils, destroy the critically needed essential fatty acids, which are required for arterial and heart health, whereas organic butter is protective. Furthermore, margarine, hydrogenated oils, and partially hydrogenated oils are known to specifically raise cholesterol levels.

In the cause of circulatory diseases Bicknell implicates two foods: white flour, depleted of all nutrients and loaded with chlorinated toxins, and hydrogenated/partially hydrogenated oils, for instance, margarine and deep frying oils. In order to avoid or reverse heart and arterial disease all such foods must be strictly avoided. When dining in restaurants, make clear to your server not to bring the bread basket. Have the server clear all crackers from the table. Do not eat pasta. Never eat white bread. Avoid all sweets or foods prepared with flour. Buy only coarse unprocessed whole grains and whole grain cereals. If cereal must be consumed, use only oat bran or brown rice cereals, perhaps for a wheat-based cereal Red River Cereal (coarse wheat, flax seed, and rye). Remember, all white flour is gassed, either with chlorine or bromine, both of which are unforgiving in their toxicity. Heart and arterial diseases were essentially unknown prior to the introduction of white flour and margarine. These are killer foods. Avoid them at all costs.

There are other food additives which are of concern, for instance, food dyes. One of these dyes, tartrazine, is a major cause of allergic reactions. In Europe this is known as E102, while in North America it is represented by FD & C Yellow #5 or, simply, tartrazine. It is an orange or even yellow-greenish dye commonly used to give an even color to orange juice as well as in coloring drugs. According to J. A. Trimbrell, in his book, *Introduction to Toxicology*, tartrazine is highly toxic, especially to children. It is a direct cause of wild and agitated behavior in children, including purposeless actions. It also causes hives and rashes. What's more, it is toxic to the lungs and may result in asthma reactions. The fact is it is a primary cause of such attacks.

Look carefully on labels for Yellow Dye #5, artificial colors, and/or tartrazine. Avoid foods and beverages which contain this dye. Other food additives which may damage the body include MSG, sodium benzoate, polysorbate 80, artificial flavors, propellants, stabilizers, emulsifiers, anti-caking agents, chlorine and bromine dioxide (used to bleach flour and rice), aspartame, saccharin, and sucralose.

Think about it. All the aforementioned substances are "artificial." Why would anyone eat or drink artificial foods, which, clearly, are incapable of sustaining life? The early research proves this. When diets were artificially created, containing all the known necessary nutrients, the test animals fared poorly and, in fact, died prematurely. When, instead, whole foods were fed, the animals thrived. There is no need for further proof. Synthetic substances made from artificial compounds, particularly food additives, are unfit for human consumption.

Caffeine: chemical irritant

Caffeine is destructive to the nerves. It offers no health benefits. This is a chemical irritant, which distresses the nerves. It is the nerves which largely control blood pressure. What's more, caffeine depletes nutrients, including magnesium. It is magnesium which helps maintain muscle relaxation. A lack of this mineral causes spasticity of the muscles as well as hyper-irritability of the nerves. Magnesium depletion from the heart greatly increases the risks for heart disorders, including angina, coronary artery disease, congestive heart failure, mitral valve prolapse, and sudden death. Low magnesium levels are clearly associated with an increased risk for high blood pressure.

It is possible to determine if people are coffee drinkers. The ruddiness of the skin, the clamminess, the nervous agitation, the tense appearance: all are telltale. Perhaps one of the greatest signs is the facial pores. Enlarged facial pores are a clear signal of magnesium deficiency. Often, the number of cups of coffee drunk can be predicted by the degree of facial pore enlargement.

Food and chemical allergy: possible factors

Toxic reactions to foods or food-borne chemicals, as well as beverages, can raise blood pressure. One mechanism is the role allergic reactions play in blood clotting. Such reactions create inflammation, which may lead to thickening of the blood. In other words, the allergic reactions cause inflammation within the bloodstream, contributing to high blood pressure. Or, it causes the release of chemicals, which cause inflammation in the heart and/or arteries, which can also raise it. Regardless the cure is simple: avoid the offending agent and reverse the inflammation with naturally occurring antiinflammatory agents.

It may be difficult to determine the precise agent, which is responsible for the inflammation. One method is a specialized blood test, known as the Food Intolerance Test. This is a research-grade test, so it is only available at one laboratory in the United States. The test checks for some 230 foods and food additives, virtually all the important ones in the American diet. It is highly accurate, that is far more accurate than any test available in the typical allergist's office. Any doctor can order this test, although it requires a special type of preservative-free blood tube. For more information regarding this test call 1-800-243-5242. Foods and beverages, which through allergic reactions typically cause thickening of the blood, include allergic reactions to seafood, wheat, rye, malt, corn, sugar, potatoes, baker's yeast, and dozens of others. This is the most accurate food allergy test available, highly valuable for the reversal of chronic disease.

There are numerous allergy tests. The Food Intolerance Test is perhaps the only one which consistently provides reliable results, which are clinically applicable.

Potent estrogens: a woman's doom

In susceptible individuals hormone pills cause high blood pressure. This is particularly true of the potent animal-source estrogen known as Premarin. Such hormonal products are a proven cause of blood clots, arterial damage, strokes, and heart attacks. With these high risks why would anyone take them? Potent estrogen-based pills have been associated with a wide range of diseases. The typical pharmaceutical pills are being scrutinized due to their highly toxic actions. The government has even condemned their use due to the associated increased risk in serious diseases, including Alzheimer's, stroke, and heart attack. Countless women in the Western world have died prematurely because of these drugs. They have done the women no good: only harm. Perhaps in some instances such estrogens may have provided relief, that is from symptoms such as hot flashes. Yet, at what cost—premature death from Alzheimer's disease, Parkinson's disease, multiple sclerosis, autoimmune disorders, stroke, heart attack, blood clots, and hypertensive crises? The fact is the cost has been unfathomable.

Premarin is particularly vile. No doctor should prescribe it. This is mare's estrogen, derived from the urine of pregnant horses. The horses are artificially inseminated and then held in tight quarters. They are force-fed, usually prefabricated feed. They frequently become ill and suffer from infections. The infectious material becomes deposited in the urine. There is no way to sterilize it. Thus, when the drug is made the septic components are included.

By taking Premarin a person gets much more than urinary estrogens: there are also viruses, bacteria-like organisms, chemical toxins, antibiotic residues, and worse than even these, neurotropic germs. The neurotropic germs, which are associated with mad cow syndrome, are derived from the feed. These cause permanent brain damage. This may explain a devastating finding: the fact that Premarin users are over three times more likely to develop Alzheimer's disease, which is a mad cow-like syndrome, than the norm. The fact is throughout the Western world there are tens of thousands of individuals who have developed senility diseases largely as a result of this drug. Avoid horse urine estrogens like you would avoid the plague.

Chlorine: death in a glass?

The fact that chlorine is toxic is indisputable. Yet, people often think nothing of the most dangerous source of chlorine of all: tap water.

Tap water contains dangerous amounts of chlorine as well as various chlorinated derivatives. All such substances are toxic to the cardiovascular system, that is the arterial walls and heart. It was Joseph M. Price, M. D., author of *Coronaries, Cholesterol, Chlorine*, who described the connection. In his book he documents how this noxious chemical directly damages the arteries as well as the heart.

Some might say, "Chlorine kills germs, so it must be good for us." While this is true regarding epidemic diseases, that is typhus, cholera, hepatitis, and similar water-borne diseases, this does not exempt chlorine from a simple fact: all forms of this chemical are toxic.

Chlorine is a cellular poison. It readily damages cells by causing direct damage to its membranes as well as genetic material. Contrast this to cholesterol, which, in fact, is a preservative of the cell membrane. Cholesterol helps rebuild cell membranes; chlorine destroys them. This is why Price dedicated an entire chapter to the issue: The Cholesterol Theory. Notice the use of the term, theory. The fact is Price summarizes the research, confirming that there is no proven link between dietary cholesterol and heart disease. He describes this molecule's rightful place in the body:

Cholesterol is a fatty (lipid) which occurs in all animal cells and which is *essential to life*. It is needed by the body as a chemical starting point for many needed compounds. For example, the vital steroidal hormones, which include the basic male and female sex hormones, can be made only from cholesterol. The human brain itself contains a very high percentage of cholesterol.

What's more, after a thorough review of the literature Dr. Price makes a bold statement: "dietary consumption of fat bears little relationship to the development of atherosclerosis."

It makes no sense that cholesterol is the cause. Consider the many peoples, such as the French, Greeks, Turks, and the Inuit who consume cholesterol-rich foods liberally. In some regions the Chinese and Japanese consume significant amounts, as do, particularly, the Mongolians. Yet, in each of these cultures heart disease is rare. Clearly, now, the cholesterol theory is debunked. Price described an additional compelling fact: in the United States prior to the 1930s heart disease was utterly rare. The mass chlorination of the water began in the 1930s and 40s.

Chlorine is one of the most potent oxidizing agents known. This is how it damages the heart and arteries. What's more, when water is chlorinated a vast number of noxious compounds are created: these substances are known as chlorinated hydrocarbons. The fact is chlorinated hydrocarbons are among the most toxic substances known. Such chemicals are potent oxidizing agents. They are also powerful carcinogens. There is no question that if sufficient amounts of such substances enter the bloodstream, damage will occur.

Everyone knows that common chlorine, in the form of bleach, is ultra-poisonous. It is a skull-and-crossbones-like material. The precautions for using it are extensive. Would it be any different when ingesting it in drinking water? Here too precautions must be taken, that is to avoid drinking such chemically-tainted water. There is another concern: shower and bath water. Here, a person is exposed to chlorine in two ways: through direct absorption through the skin and inhalation of the gas, that is from evaporation. Such an exposure can be even more damaging than direct consumption. This emphasizes the need for water purification. The fact is with the proper equipment some 99.9% of the chlorine can be removed. This is critical, particularly for individuals with a vulnerability to heart disease and cancer.

Chlorine is one of the most potent carcinogens known. It must be removed from the water at all costs. A high grade water purification system is now available. Known as LifeSource, this is the only state-of-the-art system available. The company is registered with the Water Quality Association and is the main innovator in the field. Lifesource specializes in whole-home units. For more information talk to a sales representative at: 1-800-992-3997. This is the most dependable and effective unit available, which is backed by reliable research.

The role of chlorine and various chlorinated toxins in heart disease, as well as cancer, is indisputable. Chlorine is a toxic chemical, and in high doses it irritates and, ultimately, damages the arteries. Price proved in his experiments the scope of the damage. In experiments on chickens he found that the addition of chlorine to the water led to massive arterial damage, including the formation of the typical plaques of human disease. The experiments were repeated, producing the same results.

As part of the treatment plan for high blood pressure and/or heart disease the water that an individual bathes in and drinks should be decontaminated. As a result the individual's health will remain at the highest possible level. Chlorine is a deadly poison. Its intake must be avoided. Certainly, it should never be used for cleaning food or vegetables. There are far safer options. For instance, the Oreganol may be used. Simply add a few drops, along with a safe surfactant, to the soaking water. Let it sit for a few moments, then rinse. Or, use the pre-mixed OregaSpray. This can be safely sprayed on all foods. The fact is it is fully edible. It both cleanses and decontaminates, and, since it is made from food-grade spice oils, it is completely non-toxic. Its regular use will largely prevent food poisoning. In tests OregaSpray was found to kill common food-borne molds, and it is also antibacterial. OregaSpray can be sprayed in the air for decontamination. It is highly effective in neutralizing the ill effects of chemical fumes, including chlorine and sulfur gas as well as cigarette smoke. Sprayed into the air it helps unplug clogged sinuses. It is also effective as a spray on damaged skin as well as burns and wounds. It even kills drug-resistant germs. Thus, it is ideal for hospitals and doctor's offices as well as simply the home. This spray has hundreds of uses. A partial list of the uses of OregaSpray includes for cleaning the skin and hands, as a nursery or air spray, to cleanse the air of odors, as a deodorant, to kill germs in the rest room, to repel biting insects, as a natural pesticide, to cleanse the air in a sick room, as a spray for pets, as a kitchen surface cleaner, to neutralize allergens, as a toothbrush or dental spray, and as a throat spray. It is also an excellent spray for skin disorders, including fungal conditions, as well as wounds. To purchase OregaSpray check finer health food stores or call 1-800-243-5242.

Chapter 4

Food, Fat, and More

Certain foods, as well as nutritional supplements, help heal the heart and arteries. The most powerful of these will be described in this chapter. Many such foods are fat-rich. While this is contrary to what many people believe the rationale for their use will be described. What's more, misconceptions about food will be dispelled. The truly harmful foods will be revealed, while those which can help heal the tissues and organs are emphasized.

Cholesterol is not the issue

Don't waste your time focusing on cholesterol. It has little if anything to do with high blood pressure. Cholesterol is a critical substance, which is required by every cell in the body. A high cholesterol level rarely causes high blood pressure. In any case the diet in this book will help normalize the cholesterol levels, as will the supplements. It is important to also realize that drugs which lower cholesterol also destroy vitamin E and coenzyme Q-10, both of which are critical for maintaining normal blood pressure.

A moderately high cholesterol is of no concern. There has developed a kind of cholesterol paranoia. Here, people worry about their levels, even if they are borderline high. The fact is a moderately high cholesterol level rarely increases the risk for disease.

Incredibly, peoples' cholesterol levels have become the topic of conversation. People should stop focusing on this and instead concentrate on a healthy diet. The diet in this book will lower cholesterol levels in a natural way: but not too low. A level of between 175 and 200 is ideal. There is only a concern when levels rise above 250, and even then there is no need to panic. Simply eliminating the refined carbohydrates will cause it to drop.

Yet, levels which are exceedingly low are, in fact, dangerous. This demonstrates the fallacy of forcibly lowering this substance. The fact is cholesterol levels below 160 are associated with a high risk for cancer, heart disease, and neurological disorders as well as sudden death.

A persistently high cholesterol in women over 40 warns of a thyroid imbalance. Simply boosting thyroid function brings the cholesterol to normal. Thyroset is a thyroid-balancing supplement made with a high grade of deep northern Pacific kelp. The kelp plus associated herbs and nutrients greatly boosts thyroid function in a natural way. Thus, it is useful for both hyper- and hypothyroid conditions. The point is forcibly lowering cholesterol levels with potent drugs is never the answer. Rather, the cause must be treated, so that the cholesterol level can be normalized.

Medical studies, notably the PROSPER vascular risk evaluation, prove that the regular use of cholesterol-lowering drugs greatly increases the incidence of cancer. In *The Consultant* Steven Horvitz, D.O. notes that cholesterol is absolutely critical for tissue repair. He hypothesizes that denying the body this essential substance results in the growth of cancers. David Nash, M.D., in the same article attempts to oppose Horvitz's concerns by claiming that while cholesterol is a tissue building substance, drugs which lower this substance "will improve the lives of many..." Yet, how could this be so? Is a three-fold increased risk of cancer and a six-fold increase in violent death—as are caused by such drugs—an improvement? Is the constant need to monitor liver enzymes, that is due to concerns of drug toxicity, a lifestyle benefit?

The point is people should quit concentrating on cholesterol. It is not a major issue. It is a reparative agent. It is high, largely because there is toxicity and/or tissue damage. In other words, cholesterol, which is an antioxidant, is produced to ward off toxicity. This damage, which is creating such a stress reaction, must be addressed. Through this the root cause can be treated. Much of this damage is due to infection.

Natural cures for high cholesterol

When the infection is eradicated, the cholesterol levels become normalized. This eradication can be advanced through the regular use of Oreganol P73, that is the edible oil of wild oregano. What's more, there are natural substances, which lower cholesterol. These include crude red sour grape, cumin extract, wild northern kelp, and garlic concentrate. All these substances are found in Cholestamin. Regarding the latter the combination of these ingredients offers three mechanisms of actions for lowering cholesterol: the halting of oxidative damage in the arteries, improvement of bile synthesis in the liver, and the direct effect upon cholesterol absorption. The wild kelp bolsters thyroid function, which causes cholesterol to be metabolized.

Plus, Cholestamin contains natural chromium, a well known cholesterol-lowering agent. Yet, ultimately, it is a radical change in diet, which has the greatest impact. All processed foods must be strictly avoided and/or restricted. In some individuals, particularly those with sluggish metabolism and/or thyroid disorders, even healthy foods, for instance, high carbohydrate foods, such as brown rice, yams, potatoes, and whole grain bread, must be avoided. The diet varies for each individual. For further information see *How to Eat Right and Live Longer* as well as the recipe section of this book.

Cholesterol is used as a sealant. On a daily basis the body produces vast amounts for protective purposes. There can only be one reason that the body makes this: to protect and build tissues. Forcibly lowering it proves disastrous. Every day the liver alone produces the equivalent of a dozen or two dozen eggs-worth of this molecule. Under stress even greater amounts are produced. Cholesterol is required for dozens of critical, in fact, lifesaving functions, including the synthesis of nerve sheaths, hormones, neurotransmitters, digestive aids (i.e. bile), and cell wall components. Every cell requires a daily supply of cholesterol for survival. In fact, this substance is direly needed by the body: the more the better. A cholesterol-rich diet, such as the type of diets followed by the Masai, the Yemeni villagers, the mountain-dwelling Turks, and the Caucasus Russians, is directly tied to a longer life.

Food should be eaten due to its nutritional quality, as well as its truly natural status, not in relation to cholesterol content. Do not forcibly remove cholesterol from the body. Doing so greatly increases the chances for sudden death. Any forcible removal will result in organ damage. There is no preventive benefit in forcibly lowering cholesterol. Rather, the cholesterol level can be readily normalized, just by changing the diet. *How to Eat Right and Live Longer* (Knowledge House 2001) is based upon an easy-to-follow system of eating, which is ideal for naturally lowering cholesterol levels.

CASE HISTORY (as found in the book):

Mr. J., a 55-year-old corporate executive, suffered from a high cholesterol level, despite strict dieting. He had tried a low-fat diet rich in beans and rice, to no avail, in fact, his cholesterol level increased. I put him on my diet in *How to Eat Right and Live Longer,* rich in natural healthy fats and oils, along with the appropriate fruits and vegetables. Within two months his cholesterol level dropped nearly 100 points, his lowest level ever.

People with heart disease fear the intake of cholesterol. So do diabetics. Such people have been trained to think this way. Why was heart disease so rare, that is in the 1920s and 30s, when people ate large quantities of butter, cheese, egg yolks, and beef, without giving it thought? The thinking and fretting about it, that is the fear, is more damaging than the cholesterol. There is no need to fear eating foods rich in cholesterol. Rather, their consumption should be pursued. In fact, the most long-lived of all peoples, the Caucasus Russians and the mountain-dwelling Turks, are major cholesterol eaters. The point is enjoy life.

There is nothing wrong with eating healthy and robust foods. Such foods are incapable of harming the heart or arteries. Rather, these foods nourish such organs. As is proven by the most long-lived people, including many American centenarians, there is no harm in it. How many eggs can be eaten on the all-natural fat plan—even for those with high blood pressure and heart disease? It is as many as are desired. However, they must be organic or free-range. Commercial eggs are unfit for human consumption. This is due to the types of feed given to commercial chickens. Always buy farm-fresh or free range eggs, where chickens eat either pure grains or natural forage.

The cholesterol link to high blood pressure has never been proven. In contrast, alcohol has been directly linked to this disease. All the focus is on cholesterol, while the primary perpetrators, alcohol and refined sugar, are neglected. Interestingly, alcohol destroys cholesterol. It does so by dissolving it. This may be why in some studies alcohol intake has been associated with a drop in cholesterol levels. Regarding the cells, incredibly, it dissolves their outer, that is cholesterol, coating. It also destroys the linings of the arteries and the heart muscle.

There is no evidence that naturally occurring cholesterol, such as that contained in egg yolk, beef, fish, or poultry, directly damages any tissue. Alcohol causes damage and, yet, it is prescribed. Cholesterol causes no damage and, yet, it is restricted, in fact, purged. The fact is the body uses cholesterol to repair tissues and synthesizes it for this purpose. If cholesterol is made the enemy, this will likely lead to premature death.

Fat is the issue: the right fat

Healthy fats are a required part of the diet, even for the heart and arteries. The longest lived people, who, again, are relatively free of heart disease, are fat-eaters. The fat they eat is the healthy natural type, which the heart requires. The heart requires fat in relatively large quantities. It uses it as fuel. If fat is severely restricted, the heart degenerates: so do the arteries. It was Roger Williams, Ph.D., who showed in animal studies that processed foods depleted of natural fats, in this instance, skim milk, cause arterial degeneration. Incredibly, when the animals were fed unprocessed food—pure whole milk—there was no arterial degeneration, rather, the arteries were healthy. Incredibly, the secret to the blood pressure cure is the fat content. The higher the diet is in natural fats the more vigorous will be the cure.

Fat is not the killer

There is a great deal of misinformation regarding fat. People think that by eating it they are putting their lives at risk. This is far from the truth. The fact is fat is a necessary part of the diet. It is impossible to survive without it. It is even required for the heart and arteries.

Fat, that is the natural fat found in whole foods, fights degeneration. It protects the cells of the body from metabolic decline. It is a required part of cell structure. It is critical for cellular metabolism. Purposely stripping it from the diet can never prevent disease. All it can do is cause harm.

Fat is in the food for a reason. It is a naturally occurring component—forcibly removing it disturbs the chemistry of the food. Thus, if such an altered food is consumed, it will cause disturbances. As mentioned previously this was proven by Roger Williams, famous biochemist and discoverer of pantothenic acid. Let's review his research in greater detail. Dr. Williams fed some of his animals skim milk, while feeding others whole milk. He studied the effect of these foods on arterial health. Incredibly, he found that the arteries of the whole milk-fed animals were virtually perfect, while those of the skim milk-fed animals were diseased, inflamed, and hardened.

Why corrupt nature, that is when it has been so well designed? The fact is Dr. William's research proves that there are unique attributes to whole foods. Incredibly, whole foods have in a sense their own intelligence, which, if disturbed, leads to dire consequences. Natural, that is organic, milk is a perfect food. There is no means for man to improve upon it, that is by altering its chemistry. Skim milk fails to sustain test animals, but whole milk fully does so. Is there need for any other proof that the makings of the divine source, God almighty, are irrefutable?

The Lord of the universe made much sustenance for humankind. True, there are people who fail to believe in this. Yet, regardless of beliefs all people are benefitting from these creations. They are creations which have direct curative powers. It is only a matter of taking advantage of it and avoiding any corruptions. In other words, it is critical to keep the Godly, that is true natural medicines, in their original state. Any extreme alteration will negatively effect the potency. Any corruption in the original nature of food or food-like substances will have a negative effect on health.

The fact is Dr. Williams expected that the skim milk-fed animals would suffer. A Ph.D. in nutrition he knew the value of whole unprocessed foods, such as pure whole milk, that is as a source of key nutrients. He was well aware that the skimming process would cause the loss of critical nutrients, including the fat-loving pantothenic acid. The latter is found mainly in animal foods and, in fact, is a rare substance in vegetables and/or fruit. The exception is avocado, which contains a fair amount. Pantothenic acid is highly protective for the cardiovascular system and, in fact, is required for the intracellular production of energy. Every heart and arterial cell is dependent upon it. If it is deficient, the entire cardiovascular system fails. Whole milk products, eggs, and fresh (organic) meat are the top sources of this nutrient. This is a testimony against a purely vegetable-based diet. In fact, such a diet leads to cardiovascular degeneration.

Even so, some people react negatively to milk products, even organic ones. In such individuals milk products cause a wide range of disconcerting symptoms. One way to prevent this is to take wild oregano products at the same time. To neutralize some of the toxicity or reactivity of milk products take OregaMax, which is the raw crude herb, and oil of wild oregano (P73) with any such food; sprinkle the OregaMax in yogurt or on cheese. As a result there will be a major reduction in any reactions, especially digestive symptoms. The fact is the regular intake of OregaMax and the oregano oil greatly decreases any tendencies to react to foods.

There is nothing dangerous about whole milk or whole milk products. It is how the cattle are raised and fed that is the issue, not the milk per se. Thus, pure organic milk or milk products is a health food. True, some people are allergic to milk products. However, other than this issue they are healthy foods. The fact is milk, cheese, and yogurt are among the most nutritious and well-digested foods known. Such foods, that is if organic and natural, are far more digestible than their vegetable counterparts, that is soy, nuts, and grains.

Yet, only organic milk products must be consumed. The intake of commercial milk products from cows fed commercial feeds should be strictly avoided. What's more, such cows are injected with drugs, antibiotics, and the carcinogenic Bovine Growth Hormone. A product of the Monsanto Corporation, this is a genetically-engineered poison. Eventually, it will be shown that this substance is a major cause of obesity, cancer, and other disorders, particularly in children. The government in concert with special interest groups lobbied to approve this; there is no proof of its safety. In Capital Hill Monsanto holds a number of high level lobbying positions. This is how it gains approvals, that is for unproven substances. The fact is such substances are sold merely for financial gain. Concerning this company there is no regard for the human race or this planet. Rather, Monsanto Corporation has directly contributed to the destruction of this earth as well as its inhabitants.

Monsanto was recently convicted for paying brides. Thus, it achieves its market power through corruption. The fact is evidence exists showing Bovine Growth Hormone's potential noxious effects, not only on cows but also on humans, which is why officials in Canada refused to approve it.

Recently, a batch of this genetically engineered hormone was contaminated and had to be recalled. The company refused to admit to the actual contaminant.

Since the introduction of this fabricated hormone numerous children have developed bizarre cancers. These cancers appear traceable to the consumption of commercial dairy products laced with the Monsanto hormone. From the plethora of evidence the most likely cause for these adolescent cancers is BST. The fact is this synthetic hormone is a carcinogen.

The productions of Monsanto are causing vast destruction of the environment. Its pesticides have poisoned uncountable thousands of animals as well as humans. Its genetically engineered corn has wreaked havoc globally on wildlife as well as cattle. Avoid supporting such a diabolical organization, which causes only destruction to the human race as well as this planet. Monsanto provides no environmentally beneficial substances. Rather, its creations only cause harm. The fact is anyone who supports such a company is, in fact, supporting his or her own demise.

Regardless, when consuming any milk product, a way to minimize toxicity is to add a few drops of the edible P73 Oreganol. The Oreganol is a broad-spectrum germicide and can cleanse and purge virtually any toxin. What's more, ideally, take a few drops of the Oreganol twice daily to protect the gut, since this is where most food toxicity develops. For cheese sprinkle it with the contents of OregaMax capsules.

It would be dire to attempt to live on vegetation alone. When possible, attempt to include a greater variety of foods. Shop for truly organic milk products or imported types from regions free of mad cow syndrome. This will insure a more solid nutritional status and, therefore, improved health.

Regarding overweight people there is a major issue, that is how people have been trained—to think. This thinking is that, somehow, the consumption of cholesterol-rich foods is fattening. Yet, foods rich in cholesterol are just that: edible, natural foods. In fact, they are non-fattening. Such foods are simply a part of the natural diet. There is no way natural fats can cause harm, even the naturally-occurring fats and supposedly heavy fats, for instance, the fats in beefsteak, egg yolks, or butter. The fact is a greater amount of fat develops on a person's body due to carbohydrates rather than fats.

You may try an experiment on yourself for a few days. Eat large amounts of healthy fats for a few days as the only food: egg yolks, organic butter, whole milk cheese, organic full fat cottage cheese, olives, fatty meats, fatty fish, nuts, nut butters, and seeds. Eat only these foods, no others, for, a week or two. Weigh yourself regularly and mark the results. Then, for the same amount of time eat only starches: pasta, potatoes, vegetables, fruit, yams, beans, bread, rolls, muffins, granola, and cereal. Weigh yourself regularly and mark the results. Assuredly, on the latter diet you will only gain weight, as represented by an increase in fat cells. Starch is the poor man's food in more ways than just economical.

Regarding the cause of heart disease, much has been written implicating cholesterol and saturated fat. Heart disease and high blood pressure patients, as well as diabetics, religiously avoid foods rich in such fats/lipids. This is a catastrophic error. Incredibly, this violates natural physiology. The fact is the cells of the body require fat as fuel. They thrive on it. There is no evidence of damaging effects, that is from the regular or even massive intake of naturally occurring fats. Remember Roger Williams' work: the consequences of violating nature. Don't succumb to the marketing tactics of the corporate world.

Years ago I received an order from a provincial milk board (in Canada) for my book, *How to Eat Right and Live Longer*. They claimed to be interested in the fact that I recommended milk products. The board was excited to get the book; the person ordering it seemed spirited. Months passed since I had sent it, so I called them. When they realized it was me, they became indifferent, even hostile. They said, "We have no further interest," and "were not pleased with the book."

What an incredible reaction. However, the motive behind this is easy to understand. I condemned the intake of processed milk products, especially skimmed milk. Versus whole milk the milk board earns greater income on skimmed milk; this achieves them twice the revenue. They profit from the altered milk, while selling the cream for a premium. Plus, they claim health benefits from this corrupted milk, the fallacy of which is easy to prove. As demonstrated by the eminent Roger Williams, Ph.D., such claims are bogus. The fact is the Manitoba Milk Board wanted nothing to do with my tell-it-like-it-is approach.

Natural fats can be consumed with impunity. For people with heart disorders, as well as high blood pressure, the benefits are notable. This is represented by a stronger heart, reduction in heart rhythm disturbances, stronger heart valves, greater physical strength, increased stamina, more powerful lung function, and reduction in blood pressure: all from eating larger quantities of fat. This is an incredible statement, yet it is a fact. Try it; you will find it true.

Fat is the fuel which keeps the internal organs in top condition. The cells thrive upon it. It is easy to burn, and it produces large amounts of energy. Consider the pressures on the human heart. In some people this organ may pump up to 100,000 times daily. This is a vast degree of action, which could readily exhaust even the most reliable organ. The protection of this muscle is its energy source: fat.

The holy books give mention to fat, that is as a health food in the form of whole milk, cattle, and extra virgin olive oil. This heart-health connection may be why, for instance, in the Qur'an olive oil is mentioned as a divine gift. Scientific studies demonstrate that its monounsaturated oils are an ideal fuel source for the heart. Other sources of such oils include avocados, pecans, almonds, filberts, macadamia nuts, sesame seeds, poppy seeds, pumpkin seeds, pistachios, and wild game. Lean and grass-fed beef and lamb are also good sources of such oils. The oils from these foods are ideal fuel fats, and, thus, they keep the heart muscle amply supplied with the energy it requires.

Fat is even needed for the brain. Recently, an early 20th century diet for epilepsy has been revived. Called the Ketogenic Diet this is, essentially, a severely carbohydrate- and sugar-restricted diet, which is particularly high in natural fats. The fats largely come from saturated and monounsaturated sources. There is little or no carbohydrate on this diet, much like the Atkin's plan. On this diet the vast majority of epileptics go into remission, a remarkable achievement. Such results can be largely attributed to the positive actions of this diet on the pancreas as well as the liver. These are the organs which control blood sugar, and blood sugar disorders are directly tied to epilepsy. It is also due to the fat that certain fats and lipids, notably cholesterol and phospholipids, directly fuel the brain.

The powers of olive oil

Without doubt, olive oil increases life span. In all societies where it is a staple people live longer, and they are relatively free of killer diseases, that is versus their Western counterparts. In particular, the incidence of heart disease, as well as high blood pressure, is lower in regular olive oil users. Thus, this fat acts as a kind of preventive, even cure, for this condition.

Extra virgin olive oil is a preservative. This is how it acts within the tissues, that is it preserves cellular health. It helps prevent the cells from degenerating. This will help keep the tissues as youthful as possible, while helping to prevent degeneration.

In ancient Greece the olive tree largely grew wild. The Greeks discovered that the wild oil was particularly medicinal. They used it to purge the body of toxins. Applied to the skin it helped cleanse it and kept it beautiful. Hippocrates describes its powers when taken internally in reversing skin diseases and, topically, in healing skin ulcers. Apparently, it was also used as an aid to childbirth, that is as a lubricant.

Today, therapists are very familiar with its medicinal actions. Even though it is a thick oil extra virgin olive oil is ideal for rubbing into the skin for reversing inflammation and pain. The combination of this oil plus spice oils, that is the Oreganol P73, is a potent topical rub for any pain syndrome. The ideal form for massage is the P73 SuperStrength Oreganol. Research determined that the active ingredient of Oreganol, wild oil of oregano spice, possesses morphine-like properties. Thus, the olive oil-oregano oil combination is the ideal emollient for arthritis, muscle aches, tendonitis, carpal tunnel syndrome, synovitis, sprains, and similar joint/muscular diseases.

Olive oil feeds the heart. It improves the pumping ability of the heart, preventing or warding off its decline. The heart must receive fatty fuels on a regular basis. The routine intake of extra virgin olive oil fills this need. What's more, although the mechanism is largely unknown, extra virgin olive oil prevents hardening of the arteries as well as hypertension.

Coconut and palm oil: heart-healthy

For decades only vegetable oils have been promoted as heart-healthy. In particular, margarine has been heavily touted. In fact, millions of Americans switched from butter (and even olive oil) to various vegetable-based oils—corn oil, salad oil, margarine, Canola oil, soy oil, etc.—all to their detriment.

Coconut and palm oils were once common additives in processed foods. Then, in the 1980s a massive campaign was directed against them, which included full-paged ads in major newspapers warning of deleterious effects. The campaign was financed by the soybean industry. Legitimate health concerns were not the source. It drove the coconut and palm oil sources in this country out of business. As a result, incredibly, Americans' health suffered. This is because the relatively digestible and healthy tropical oils, which had been safely used by people for centuries, were replaced by the highly polyunsaturated vegetable oils. This is detrimental, because the polyunsaturates are pro-inflammatory. The rise in heart disease is directly tied to the increased intake of such oils, while, for instance, in Sri Lanka, where coconut oil and palm oil are staples, the incidence of heart disease is incredibly low—perhaps the lowest in the world. The fact is in their pure state such "tropical oils are heart-healthy, never damaging.

Coconut and palm oils contain special fatty acids known as medium chain triglycerides. These fatty acids are ideal for the heart muscle: it uses them as fuel. They are easily absorbed and non-toxic. They fail to promote inflammation. What's more, they contain substances, notably lauric acid, which strengthen immunity.

A heart healthy tropical oil has recently become available. Known as CocaPalm, this spice oil-fortified plant oil is ideal for use in cooking and baking. It can only help the health of the heart. It will not harm it. Regions where coconut oil is extensively consumed, such as Sri Lanka and Malaysia, have among the lowest incidence of heart disease known. This is the original spiced coconut oil, rich in aromatic and antioxidant spice oils. These oils help prevent dangerous free radicals from forming during cooking. Thus, cocapalm is the ideal type of oil for deep frying, sautéing, or basting. It also makes a wonderful spread, which can replace butter (See appendix A).

Crude cold-pressed sesame oil (Sesam-E): major power source

This is the ideal dietary oil for heart health. This is because it is rich in substances which prevent the degeneration of such organs. While coconut and palm oils play a significant role it is cold-pressed sesame oil which is the most unique. This is because of its rich profile of antioxidants, which help support the health of the heart and arteries. Coconut and palm oils provide fuel fats. Palm oil also provides vitamin E and beta carotene. Sesame is rich in its own forms of antioxidants: sesamol and sesamin. It also contains a considerable amount of vitamin E.

In regions where sesame is a staple there is a longer life span than in regions where it is unknown. Surely, the potent sesame oil antioxidants are the major reason for this finding.

Crude sesame oil helps build strength, including the powers and strength of the internal organs. It contains a powerful group of substances, including antioxidants, which are up to ten times more powerful than vitamin E. Thus, when regularly consumed crude cold-pressed sesame oil, that is the Sesam-E, replaces any need for vitamin E supplements. For an ideal crude and natural vitamin E supplement combine a few tablespoons of both the Sesam-E and the Pumpkinol daily. What's more, the crude natural vitamin E is far superior in potency and healing powers to the commercial, that is semi-synthetic, variety.

Commercial sesame oil fails to offer this benefit. Largely, it is either heat extracted or toasted. This destroys much of its medicinal value. Plus, it is made from commercially raised sesame seeds versus the more primitive sources. In contrast, Sesam-E is a non-commercial sesame oil, which is truly cold-pressed. This is the original crude cold-pressed oil from the primitive regions of Asia Minor. The extraction is via the original generations-old method, all from a virtual wilderness region. No chemicals or pesticides are used. It is this type of sesame oil, which offers the greatest medicinal powers. What's more, it is free of genetically engineered components. Sesam-E has an exceptionally rich taste. To buy or order this luscious and nutritionally rich oil check high quality health food stores or call 1-800-243-5242. This oil may also be viewed at various Web sites. Enter in the search engine, Sesam-E and/or North American Herb & Spice. It is a rare oil. Shortages may occur.

For the reversal of any blood pressure disorder and/or heart defect the regular intake of Sesam-E is crucial. This is confirmed by the latest science. There are a number of substances in this oil, which lower blood pressure. The study, reported to the American Heart Association's Society of Hypertension, determined that sesame oil alone normalized blood pressure. Conducted by Dr. D. Sankar some 320 people with high blood pressure were studied. However, these were far from normal cases. Rather, they were people with drug-resistant high blood pressure. In virtually all cases as a result of merely adding the oil to the diet the blood pressure was significantly reduced, with results being noticed in less than a month. A mere tablespoon or two of the oil was sufficient to cause a reduction. This may explain the low incidence of this disorder in regions where sesame products, such as tahini and sesame oil, are a staple. Incredibly, these benefits were seen, even in people who used the oil in cooking. Thus, for people with high blood pressure if foods are to be cooked in oil, use sesame oil. Ideally, Sesam-E is the most healthful choice.

This indicates that by replacing commercial cooking oils with the Sesam-E there is a benefit, since in this study sesame oil replaced all other oils. When cooked, the typical vegetable oils are oxidized. When ingested, this oxidized oil causes internal damage, including oxidative damage of the heart and arteries.

Thus, for those with heart and arterial disease the ideal cooking oils are Sesame-E and cocapalm. The cocapalm is superior to regular coconut oil. This is because it is infused with antioxidant spice oils. A buttery yellow, it contains oils of wild oregano and rosemary as well as oils of turmeric, fenugreek, and coriander. These oils have a high antioxidant profile on ORAC testing. Thus, cocapalm is more stable to heat than plain coconut oils.

Regarding Sesam-E there is another benefit: a high gamma tocopherol content. This is the antioxidant form of vitamin E, rarely available in the typical vitamin E supplement. The fact is gamma tocopherol, as found in Sesam-E, is an effective preventive agent against cancer. Yet, it may provide an even more compelling action, that is in the treatment of this disease. According to Brigelious-Flohe, in her summary article on vitamin E in the *American Journal of Clinical Nutrition*, such forms of vitamin E are capable of causing cancer cell death. Thus, for general health a teaspoon daily of Sesam-E is advised.

The importance of protein

The heart is a muscle, while the arteries are connective tissue. Animal foods contain certain nutrients, which nourish these organs, notably amino acids, carnitine, vitamin B_{12}, folic acid, taurine, riboflavin, and pantothenic acid. If these nutrients are lacking, the heart and arteries can degenerate. Thus, nutritional deficiency damages the circulatory system.

Ultimately, strict vegan and/or vegetarian diets offer little if any protection against high blood pressure. There may be a temporary benefit, that is from halting the intake of processed foods. Yet, eventually, if the diet is too strict, the heart and arteries suffer. In fact, ultimately, as a result of the prolonged adherence to such a diet these organs degenerate. What's more, certainly, such diets are of little if any value in protecting the heart. In fact, these diets cause damage to the heart muscle. This is because the heart muscle thrives on fatty fuels, and a strict vegan/vegetarian diet may be devoid of these.

The heart muscle requires fat as fuel. If it is denied fatty fuels, it degenerates. For optimal health of this organ fatty fuels must be routinely supplied. For vegans to a certain degree this danger can be minimized by the regular intake of avocados and olives as well as heavy oils, such as extra virgin olive oil, black seed oil, and cold-pressed sesame oil. The intake of specialized foods, such as the protein and fatty-acid-rich bee pollen and, particularly, royal jelly, i. e. the Royal Oil, would also help diminish the risks. The fact is in vegans a teaspoonful of Royal Oil daily significantly reduces the risk for diet-induced heart damage.

It is true that the elimination of processed food aids the body, and this is achieved by strict vegetarian diets. However, even with processed foods a variety of heart-supporting food sources are consumed: meat, milk products, and eggs. With vegetarianism, and, particularly, veganism, the diet is inevitably restricted of fats, particularly the rich animal fats. In some instances animal products are completely eliminated from the diet. This diet violates normal physiology.

If the physiology of the body is violated, there are consequences. The fact is the tissues can be destroyed. In particular, the lack of B_{12} alone leads to tissue destruction, especially in the heart and arteries. This is due to the accumulation of the highly toxic compound, homocysteine.

In particular, vegan diets lead to muscular tissue damage especially of the heart. The fact is vegans commonly suffer from muscular diseases. Their diets are unavoidably incomplete. They fail to receive the nutrients they need to maintain the health of the muscular tissues as well as the bones. In fact, on such diets, the bones may rapidly degenerate. This may result in spontaneous fractures.

The heart is a muscular tissue. As a result of the vegan diet it is readily destroyed. Even so, vegans may be able to modulate the damage to a degree. This is through, for instance, the regular intake of easy-to-digest vegetable protein sources such sprouts and spouted nuts. Yet, this alone will not fully prevent the damage, which will develop due to the lack of essential amino acids. However, ultimately, unless the diet is modified brain, heart, spinal cord, arterial, and nerve damage will occur.

The vegan diet also leads to the destruction of another critical organ: the liver. I have seen numerous cases of liver damage in vegans, in fact, outright cirrhosis. The latter is a form of permanent liver damage, that is scarring of the liver tissue. Thus, as a result of a vegan diet permanent liver damage will result.

The liver thrives on protein. It is an animal tissue, which requires a certain amount of animal-source food. When denied the appropriate protein-based substances, that is the essential amino acids, which are found mainly in animal food, as well as the key cellular refueling agent, carnitine. the liver degenerates. This degeneration begins within as little as a month of a highly restrictive diet. If this degeneration is not halted, that is by the feeding of animal-source proteins, permanent damage will occur. This is known as cirrhosis of the liver, and it is due largely to severe amino acid deficiency. What's more, notoriously, the vegan diet is high in starch. In most individuals this leads to fatty liver, which accelerates this organ's degeneration.

On a vegan diet it is impossible to provide the liver with its ideal amino acid and vitamin needs. As a result organ damage is inevitable. Nor can the brain be properly nourished, nor can any other organ, including the thyroid and adrenals. Some of this may be prevented by the regular intake of sprouts and sprouted seeds, as well as crude royal jelly extracts such as Royal Oil and/or Royal Power. Yet, even so, B_{12} will be lacking, and this is direly needed by all cells.

The elimination of animal protein from the diet can be destructive. This is particularly true regarding people of northern European ancestry. The fact is, ultimately, disease will result.

It is understandable why people avoid animal products, since farming practices are so bizarre. For the treatment of high blood pressure and heart disease this is the opposite of what is desired. Inevitably, vegetable-based diets are high in carbohydrates. Yet, though often it is a sincere effort to preserve health and avoid toxicity, incredibly, in the use of the circulatory system strict or total avoidance of animal-source food leads to tissue damage. The organs which will endure the greatest damage includes the heart, arteries, liver, kidneys, bone marrow, bones, joints, adrenals, thyroid, spinal cord, and brain. Due to the increase in sugar and starch intake the blood may become sticky. This may result in blood clots, even strokes and heart attacks. This is particularly true of people with low thyroid function. Here, a vegan type diet can actually cause blood clots.

High blood pressure patients should not follow a vegan diet. Nor should anyone with liver or kidney disease. Like the liver the kidneys require a regular supply of amino acids derived from animal protein. What's more, animal foods provide salts which the blood vessel system, as well as the heart and kidneys, desperately need. The salt helps keep the circulatory system in ideal condition, maintaining normal blood volume.

No human can digest grass, in fact, even the digestion of plant foods, such as beans, soy, nuts, and lentils, is difficult. What a dire, as well as destructive, process it would be, that is for the human to attempt to gain dietary protein exclusively from vegetation. The fact is vegetables and fruit are an accent to the diet; they are cleansing and refreshing. They are never meant as a source of protein, at least not for human physiology.

It is much easier to digest, for instance, organic turkey or chicken than lentils or beans. The amino acids from the meat sources are more readily absorbed than those from the beans, nuts, or lentils, and, thus, such amino acids directly nourish the tissues, including the brain.

For vital energy it is important to at least occasionally eat animal foods. Rather, in the case of the treatment for high blood pressure the consumption of such foods must be vigorous. This is because the circulatory tree thrives on healthy animal foods, especially animal fats. Thus, for people with high blood pressure, who restrict animal foods, it is important to increase the intake of this category. As an alternative avocados and nuts help, but they fail to fully replace the powers of animal foods, which are rich in novel substances, such as pantothenic acid, vitamin B_{12}, folic acid, taurine, and carnitine, which combat this disease. Thus, it is crucial to increase the intake of healthy organic sources of meat. If not, at least the individual must eat healthy/organic milk products, yogurt, and eggs.

What a person eats is a matter of choice. This is no attempt to impose any dictates. Rather, it is merely an attempt to provide guidance, so that catastrophes will be avoided. For individuals of Western origin, that is European, Scottish, English, German, etc., a purely vegetable-based diet can be catastrophic. Thus, the issue is a highly restrictive diet can harm the individual.

Many vegans, as well as vegetarians, are exceedingly deficient in amino acids. A lack of amino acids causes damage to the internal organs. This damage can be avoided. Merely by adopting modest measures, such as the inclusion of a small amount of animal food in the diet.

Vegan diets are particularly dangerous for babies, toddlers, children, and teenagers. Here, tissue destruction is inevitable. Yet, this damage could be also prevented by minor modifications in the diet. The fact is unless critical amino acids are consumed in the form of healthy animal proteins the developing body will endure change, much of it permanent. This damage will be suffered largely by the liver and the brain. With the liver the consequence will be cirrhosis. With the brain it will be its death, as well as the death of the cells of the spinal cord. Why cause the self harm, that is if it can be avoided? The fact is regarding a more balanced diet there is a guarantee: if a strict vegan introduces healthy animal foods into the diet, his/her health will dramatically improve.

The first food a human consumes in its most vulnerable and pure state is of animal origin: from a woman's breast or the udder of an animal. The fact is, rather than soybeans or legumes, the human digestive system is fully geared to digest fresh meat, egg albumin, and fresh milk, cheese, etc.

When physiologists measure the digestibility of protein, they find a compelling fact: grains and legumes are difficult to digest, whereas fresh animal foods, that is whole milk, yogurt, eggs, poultry, and beef, are readily digested. If vegetables are supposedly the natural food, that is as a protein source, why does the human have aggressive front teeth—incisors and bicuspids—that is for the tearing of flesh? Why does a human being have a stomach acid capable of digesting even bone—with a pH of nearly 1.0—that is unless he/she is supposed to eat meat? Surely, such a potent acid secretion, capable of digesting the hand off a man: surely this isn't for mere salad vegetables.

Without at least some degree of intake of animal protein human organs degenerate. Without a reasonable intake of vitamin B_{12}, which is found mainly in meat products and to a lesser degree in eggs and milk, the brain cells degenerate. These are immutable facts, and there are no exceptions. A strict vegan diet should be avoided, that is unless as a therapy for specific diseases such as cancer. Yet, even here such a diet should be used therapeutically short-term, certainly no longer than a year or two. Any period longer than this will assuredly lead to brain cell damage as well as heart and arterial disease.

True, today regarding the safety of meat there are numerous issues. If you are concerned about the health of the meat, always cook it with spices. What's more, milk and eggs from organic sources would suffice to fill the protein needs, that is if an individual refuses to eat meat. Yet, the occasional consumption of meat, even once a month, is superior to its wholesale elimination. There are substances in meat, for instance, carnitine, taurine, essential amino acids, and iron, which are difficult to procure from any other source, even from eggs and milk.

Humans are meat eaters. From a culinary point of view meat is healthy. When prepared properly, it has a luscious and inviting taste. In fact, it is a concentrate of nutrients.

To protect against contamination meat can be marinated in vinegar, oil, and spices. Plus, take natural spice oils with any meat-containing meal. What's more, if meat is eaten with plenty of fruit and vegetables, the latter will largely cancel any negative effects. Thus, when eating meat, also eat plenty of vegetables, greens, and fruit; skip the potato.

It is well known that the meat supply, as well as the milk and eggs, particularly in the United States, has become corrupted. Yet, there are options, for instance, the consumption of truly unprocessed farm raised meats fed only on vegetation as well as truly organic meats, eggs, and milk products. There are also a wide range of fish, although certain species are so contaminated that they are virtually unfit for human consumption.

There is also the option of buying high quality bison. This animal refuses to eat anything other than fresh herbage. Bison raised exclusively upon grass/herbage is the safest possible animal food. Such bison is now available. Raised on a huge pasturage in northern Wisconsin, the North Star Bison Co., the meat of these bison is delectable and highly nutritious. This is one of the few farms which guarantees that even the finish feed before slaughtering is herbage. To contact North Star Bison and/or to order their products call 1-888-295-6332. Their Web site, which is northstarbison.com, reads that the bison is "100% grass fed" from birth to butcher.

This bison is far tastier than the commercial varieties. As most people are aware bison is far richer in protein than other types of meat. It is also exceptionally low in fat. The protein helps build strong muscle tissue. This is needed in the event of heart disease, since this organ is mostly muscle. The fact is the regular intake of bison helps strengthen the heart.

Meat, as well as milk and eggs, is a critical part of the diet. It creates vitality and supplies critical nutrients. It supplies certain nutrients, which are impossible to receive elsewhere: carnitine, taurine, lipoic acid, riboflavin, niacin, essential amino acids, preformed vitamin A, easy-to-absorb zinc, and vitamin D. The vegan diet is notoriously deficient in such nutrients, and this deficiency may result in serious disorders. This is particularly true of a deficiency of vitamin B_{12}, which is needed for the maintenance of brain tissue. The fact is this vitamin is critical for the health of brain and nerve tissue. Without it these tissues degenerate. The point is simple. If people don't fully understand what they are doing nutritionally and if they are following a restrictive diet, they can inadvertently damage themselves.

The body is dependent upon certain nutrients, and if these nutrients are strictly denied, degeneration will result. I have helped reverse this degeneration in countless individuals, who have followed restrictive diets. Because of the great degree of restrictions serious diseases developed. Then, after the individuals followed a more varied diet dramatic improvement occurred. By adding even modest amounts of fish, organic beef, organic poultry, free range/organic eggs, and organic whole milk products to the diet, disease and even premature death are halted. The best diet always includes a wide variety of foods for a wide variety of nutrients.

The human body is dependent upon strong food as well as cleansing vegetation. Consider the heart muscle. Its strength is enhanced by animal fats. Physiologists have proven that up to 90% of the fuel used by the normal heart is derived from animal fat. The fats of olive and avocado are also efficiently used, as are the fats of coconut and palm. This is largely due to their high content of saturated fats. Typical vegetable fats, such as soy and corn oil, are poorly utilized. In fact, such oils cause inflammation in the heart and arteries.

Do not be confused by this issue. Despite the standard position the fact is the primary natural fat eaters—the Inuit, Masai, Caucasus Russians, Turks, Mongolians, and numerous others—are all free of heart disease. This is true as long as they consume their natural foods, including those that are high in fat. What's more, it was the physiologist Guyton, who determined that the heart muscle is fully dependent upon dietary fat for survival. Here, experiments proved that in the normal heart 80% or more of the fuel combusted is derived from fat. This is a compelling statement: it means that in order to protect the heart from sudden failure fat must be consumed.

There is a general belief that, somehow, animal protein is stressful to the tissues. This is a vital error. The fact is animal protein is the most digestible of all types, far more so than, for instance, the protein of nuts, seeds, soy, and beans. For instance, soy is so difficult to digest that it must be fermented or at a minimum soaked. Consider nuts: how heavy they often feel on the digestion. Consider a piece of fresh organic turkey, wild fish, or natural beef; how appetizing, filling, and digestible it is.

It is true that in certain diseases animal-based foods may need to be restricted, even curtailed, for instance, cancer. Here, the blood from animal tissues may help feed the cancer. In other words, in the case of severe cancer red meat can act as a pro-carcinogen. This is in contrast to fresh fruit and vegetables, which may help halt or reverse cancer growth. However, even with cancer there is a need for protein. Ideally, the protein of, for instance, fresh organic yogurt or soured milk would suffice. As an alternative soaked nuts or soy curd may prove adequate. Regarding soy it must always be organic, since the genetically altered or commercial type is carcinogenic. What's more, a purely vegetable-based diet is lacking in key nutrients, which are needed by critical tissues such as the liver, thyroid gland, adrenals, brain, and spinal cord. B_{12} is one of the most critical of these, and a purely vegetable-based diet readily induces the deficiency, as is demonstrated by the following:

CASE HISTORY:

Ms. S. called me on the radio, complaining of a most dire symptom: complete loss of sensation in her leg to the degree that she drug it about like a stiff log. I immediately questioned her about her diet, and, as suspected, she had lived for several years on only fruits and vegetables. She had developed an extreme B_{12} deficiency with the ominous consequences of the destruction of the brain and spinal cord cells. I instructed her to immediately seek medical care, take B_{12} shots, and take the vitamin under the tongue as well as radically change the diet. She promised to do so and to include in her diet prodigious quantities of organic red meat as well as organic calves' liver. Only such an approach can regenerate her nerve cells.

This does not mean that a person must routinely eat huge quantities of meat. Today, the meat supply is less than ideal. What it means is that the total elimination of meat has ill consequences. The human body needs certain nutrients, which are concentrated in meat. Many of these nutrients are also found in milk products as well as eggs. A person can perhaps survive without meat, that is as long as there is some consumption of, for instance, eggs, milk products, and fish. However, the total elimination of all sources of animal food—meat, poultry, fish, eggs, and milk—will result in ill health. This is because, again, it violates the natural physiology of the body. The fact is such a diet encourages the development of fungal and parasitic infections, and these alone can precipitate health crises. What's more, the aforementioned foods are the primary sources in the diet of a wide range of nutrients, particularly vitamin A, vitamin D, niacin, riboflavin, pantothenic acid, zinc, coenzyme Q-10, calcium, and carnitine. Incredibly, the majority of these nutrients are essential for the function of the circulatory system.

Consider vitamin D. It is required for the utilization of calcium and magnesium; these minerals are essential for the pumping power of the heart muscle as well as the nervous control of the arteries. A lack of these minerals causes spasticity of the arteries, which may lead to both high blood pressure and heart attack. Riboflavin is required for the delivery of oxygen to the tissues. Without this critical substance the heart and arteries, as well as all other organs, degenerate.

Heart disease may largely be due to an oxygen deficiency. A lack of oxygen makes it impossible to properly utilize it, and riboflavin is essential for the cells' ability to utilize oxygen. Pantothenic acid is needed by both the heart muscle and the arteries, that is for metabolizing fuel. Without it these organs are unable to process fuel. In particular, the ability of these organs to utilize fatty acids as energy sources is compromised. This vitamin is also required for hormonal synthesis, particularly adrenal steroid production.

The adrenal steroids are the critical compounds which are needed to ward off stress and toxicity. They are also key substances for controlling blood volume and, therefore, blood pressure. What's more, the pumping power of the heart is under the influence of the adrenal steroids. Thus, an imbalance in adrenal function, which is the consequence of pantothenic acid deficiency, negatively affects the heart. This is why pantothenic acid deficiency predisposes the individual to various circulatory diseases. This is another reason to balance the vegan/vegetarian diet with high quality royal jelly.

The power of crude red sour grape

Much has been disseminated about the health benefits of flavonoids. Today, perhaps the most popular source of such flavonoids is red wine. However, there are negative effects of wine. This is why non-alcoholic sources of flavonoids are preferable. While these flavonoids, especially the red flavonoids of grapes, are cardioprotective, the alcohol is toxic. Even the alcohol in wine readily damages human tissues, notably the brain, spinal cord, red blood cells, white blood cells, and liver. Why damage one organ only to help another? The fact is a single glass of wine destroys hundreds of thousands of brain and liver cells.

Alcohol is a toxic chemical. It is the by-product of microbial fermentation. The microbes make it as a toxin: a waste product. Why humans drink it is unfathomable.

This is why unfermented sources of red grape are so valuable. A crude red sour grape powder is now available. Known as Resvital this is a truly unprocessed substance, made from sun-ripened sour grapes. Villagers pick the grapes while green and dry them in the sun until they turn a reddish brown. Then, they are pulverized by hand. The skin, seed, and pips are included, all in a convenient-to-take powder. A human trial confirms the power of this totally natural substance. Of six patients with intractable high blood pressure, all on medications, in less than six months all had their blood pressure return to normal. What's more, they all went off their medications.

Crude red grape is a rich source of resveratrol. Through a special process the resveratrol is concentrated. It is also an excellent source of chromium as well as potassium. Thus, the Resvital is a kind of natural nutritional supplement, containing vitamins and minerals completely from nature.

There is another immense benefit of this powder: blood sugar regulation. Due to its rich content of flavonoids, as well as chromium, the Resvital helps stabilize diabetes, plus it helps normalize hypoglycemia. Thus, for blood sugar regulation it is invaluable, as is demonstrated by the following:

CASE HISTORY:

Ms. T., a 55-year-old female, had a 10-year history of diabetes, which was difficult to control with medication. She suffered from a wide range of circulatory symptoms, so she decided to take the Resvital. Rapidly, the the circulatory symptoms were halted, which included cold extremities and blotches on the skin. In addition, incredibly, within three months her blood sugar normalized, apparently due to the nourishing effects of this substance upon the tissues and its high level of chromium. No one expected such results, but it was a pleasant, in fact, curative, side-effect.

Crude red grape is completely different than grape seed extract. The latter is derived from commercially raised grapes and, thus, may be contaminated with pesticides as well as fungicides. What's more, grape seed supplements are extracts. In the extraction process, chemicals are used, notably formaldehyde, methyl chloride, and hexane. All are highly toxic to the human body, as is demonstrated by the following:

CASE HISTORY:

Ms. J., a 30-year-old female, was stricken with a bizarre syndrome: the development of some 80 warts on her body. I asked her what might have provoked such a reaction. She said they developed after she took a nutritional supplement, grape seed extract, and that, previously, when she quit taking it, they disappeared. After taking it again the warts re-developed. I informed her that, as she suspected, the grape seed was the cause, but the real factor was the solvents, which are used to extract it: the grape seed itself, being a food, is harmless. Thus, rather than the grape seed extract per se it was the formaldehyde and similar solvents which were responsible. Such solvents damage the immune system of the skin cells, making them vulnerable to infection.

The Resvital is village-made, all by hand. No chemicals of any kind are applied. Nor are any solvents used in processing. It is a completely crude, unprocessed natural substance, and that is why it is so effective.

The power of pomegranate

Researchers have proven that compared to many other societies people in the Mediterranean live a long and productive life. Here, extended care facilities and nursing homes are unknown. There must be a reason for their long-lived propensities as well as for their strength in old age. Perhaps this divine fruit, this luscious and refreshing prize, the pomegranate, is a contributor. Modern science documents a possible reason: its high antioxidant profile. Of all fruit in terms of antioxidant powers pomegranate scored the highest: even higher than blueberries. Certainly, this is consistent with longevity. Pomegranate extracts exert a direct, positive action on the circulatory system. Thus, regular intake protects such critical tissues.

The long-term result of the regular use of this fruit is to live a more vital, perhaps longer, life. It is a life relatively free of the major plagues of modern civilization: heart disease, hardening of the arteries, and cancer. This fruit is specifically mentioned in the Qur'an as a blessing for the human being. A blessing would indicate a benefit. Of all citrus fruit pomegranate is the most medicinal.

Even cancer may meet its match with this fruit. This is because pomegranates are a top source of key anti-cancer substances: organic acids. The most potent of these is ellagic acid. This is a major component of this fruit. Ellagic acid is highly respected for its anti-cancer actions. Tannic and gallic acids, which are found in pomegranate in high amounts, also exhibit anti-cancer properties. These are known botanically as astringents. An astringent is a substance which has a tonic action upon the cells. Astringents act directly upon the cells, strengthening their walls as well as their internal structures. This enhances the immunity of the cells against disease. Plus, astringents, such as the organic acids found in pomegranates and similar sour fruit, are natural germicides. These substances weaken bacteria and other microbes, even destroying them. Astringents are what make tea bitter.

It is well known that a wet tea bag, placed against a skin infection, like a sty, will kill that infection. This is due to the astringents. Thus, they are a kind of herbal bitters. Pomegranate, both its juice and syrup, has a greater astringent action than virtually any other fruit, perhaps with the exception of red sour grapes. The bitter element in pomegranate is the medicinal component, which is lacking in other citrus fruit.

The chemistry of pomegranate is fascinating. Concentrated within the rind, pulp, and bark are a complex array of chemicals with great pharmacological potency. To a lesser degree these chemicals may be found in the juice. Yet, even in the juice or concentrate such chemicals exist in useful quantities. These chemicals include flavonoids, known also as proanthocyanidins, phytosterols (natural plant steroids), essential oils, and alkaloids. The latter, which may be toxic, are only found in the roots and bark.

Pomegranate cannot interfere with any medicine. However, it may reduce the need for taking such medications. In other words, by causing the person to improve there is no need to take the drugs. Rather, the fact is pomegranate reverses toxicity. Its value for the human body is far greater than any drug. The value of this medicine was discovered during the Middle Ages by Islamic physicians, who used it as an anti-parasitic. Jean Anderson's *The Nutrition Bible* describes one of this fruit's main active ingredients, ellagic acid, as an anti-carcinogen. She says that this acid, in fact, neutralizes potent cancer-causing chemicals, including aflatoxin and benzopyrene. These chemicals are such potent carcinogens that miniscule amounts can rapidly induce cancers. Yet, the acids in pomegranate readily decontaminate them. This demonstrates the impressive powers of this fruit as an antidote. The fact is the regular intake of the fruit or fruit concentrates, as well as supplements made from the seed, skin, or pulp, amount to a veritable natural cancer preventive. The regular intake of sufficient amounts may, in fact, prevent the development of cancer, perhaps entirely.

For a totally natural source of pomegranate use the Mediterranean-source Pomegranate Syrup. Free of any chemicals and pesticides this syrup is made from the original mountain-grown pomegranates found in the rocky hills of the Mediterranean. The pomegranates are boiled into a syrup, which is then used on foods or in cooking. It is ideal as an additive to salad dressings or to finish meat or poultry dishes. It is also an ideal addition to stir-fry, proving a sour taste—a great alternative for anyone who is sensitive to commercial citrus. To order Pomegranate Syrup call 1-800-243-5242.

The flavonoids: key to longevity?

Most people have heard about the French Paradox. The word paradox means that a certain trend makes little sense, that is it is the opposite of what is expected. The French eat plenty of fat, in some cases, more than many Americans. Yet, they are significantly less likely to suffer from heart disease than other Westerners. The popular media, as well as medical researchers, have attributed this protection to an unexpected source: wine. This is thought to be due not to the alcohol per se but, rather, the natural part: the red pigments, which give wine its distinctive color (and flavor). Certainly, there are benefits with these pigments. These are the flavonoids, and they possess definite medicinal properties.

Regarding wine there are also drawbacks, since alcohol is toxic and since it largely neutralizes any beneficial properties offered by the pigments. What's more, alcohol is highly addictive, while non-alcoholic sources of flavonoids, such as juices, fruit syrups, and nutritional supplements, are not. Plus, alcohol, even from wine, causes its own diseases: weakening of the heart muscle, heart muscle enlargement, that is alcoholic cardiomyopathy, high blood pressure, cirrhosis of the liver, and brain damage. The balance is against the wine, especially if it is consumed in large amounts. Thus, for the health-minded individual non-alcoholic sources of the protective compounds is the alternative.

Besides wine the French consume numerous other sources of flavonoids, for instance, fresh shellfish, a staple in this diet. Plus, the consumption of fresh herbs, a potent source of a variety of these compounds, is the norm. Dark greens of a variety of types—chervil, rosemary, oregano, mint, and sage—permeate the menus. All are exceptionally rich in flavonoids. The intake of market-fresh pungent herbs has a greater role in explaining the French Paradox than merely alcohol consumption.

Dense color implies significant medicinal actions, an observation which has been proven in the laboratory. ORAC testing has documented that the darker the pigment is the more potent the antioxidant action. The importance of color in food was first mentioned publically by Judy Kay Gray, M. S., who taught that people should select food based upon the intensity of color. What could have a greater depth in color than blackberries, which are even richer than blueberries? Black raspberries prove even higher than blackberries. Thus, black-colored berries scored significantly higher than the latter. Pomegranate came a close second. The following chart demonstrates colorful fruit and their antioxidant potential:

	ORAC values
black raspberry	164
blackberry	51
blueberry	32
pomegranate	105
cranberry	17

The power of the garlic family

This family of plants is well known for its circulatory benefits. It includes garlic, onions, shallots, and leeks. Each of these herbs is helpful in the prevention and even cure of heart disease. Each has been shown to help lower blood fat levels as well as blood pressure. Regular users of such foods have a much lower risk of heart and arterial disorders than the average.

Garlic and similar herbs contain a wide range of chemicals with medicinal properties. The majority of its powers are the result of its rich sulfur content. Sulfur is needed by the body for a wide range of functions. It is a potent germicide. It's a key compound for the function of skin, hair, and nails. What's more, it is needed for the synthesis of a key cellular component: glutathione peroxidase. This is an enzyme, which protects the cells from toxicity. The regular intake of garlic, onions, and related plants provides the body with the raw sulfur necessary for active synthesis. Through this it can keep the glutathione levels high, which means major protection for the cells.

Sulfur is readily used by the heart. Here, it is incorporated in the synthesis of cardiac glutathione. The heart, being metabolically active, generates a vast quantity of potentially toxic compounds, called free radicals. The glutathione is used to neutralize these radicals. The same is true of the arteries, which are constantly exposed to toxic compounds, for instance, through the blood, must also constantly produce glutathione. The regular intake of sulfur-rich foods, such as garlic, onion, shallots, and leeks, as well as cruciferous vegetables, such as broccoli, kale, cauliflower, and cabbage, ensures that the body's glutathione factories will be well supplied with the sulfur necessary for glutathione synthesis.

Sulfur, as found in garlic, onions, and cruciferous vegetables, helps cleanse the tissues. In the booklet, *A Prescription with 5,000 Years of History*, garlic, especially its oil, is described as a blood, as well as lymph, purifier. Say the editors: "It possesses the priceless property of cleansing whatever it contacts. Not only does it destroy the bacteria and detoxicate poisoned areas, it also exercises a positive action in toning the lymphatic cells of the body and purifying the blood stream and the intestines." Furthermore, the editors make a revelation regarding the secret to proper tissue cleansing. People have emphasized the importance of colon cleansing, that is merely purging wastes from the body, such as food toxins or other residues.

The premise of this book is that the most dire toxins of all are the germs and their residues, which accumulate in the blood and lymph. Again, to quote the editors: "It is the lymph surrounding every cell of the body that is the lurking place for waste matter and irritants. Oil of mountain-grown garlic has the invaluable capacity of penetrating the lymphatic fluid, breaking up toxic accumulation and passing it out of the body by way of the blood stream, through pores, kidneys and intestines." Of note, wild oregano oil has the same properties. Thus, to help dissolve blockages a combination spice oil extract with wild oregano and naturally extracted garlic oil would be ideal. These oils, combined with the Infla-eez, provide the ideal tissue cleansing system.

An edible oil of garlic which meets these qualifications is now available. This is the mountain-grown garlic, which is different from the commercial type. This type of garlic is of large size, plus it has a yellowish color, a sign of high sulfur content. It is fortified with wild oregano and basil oils (P73). Known as Garlex it is unique compared to commercial garlic products, because it is the cold pressed crude oil fortified with synergistic spice oils. Thus, no heat or chemicals are used in processing.

Garlex is a potent source of natural sulfur and is a combination of wild oregano extract plus mountain-derived garlic—all in the oil form. The garlic oil is made by cold-pressing. This is the most well tolerated form of garlic oil. Garlex is a natural source of the highly digestible and cleansing sulfur compounds known as sulfhydryl groups. Medically, these are also known as thiol compounds. This is the ideal way to consume dietary sulfur. Plus, as previously indicated sulfur, that is the organic forms, as found in vegetation, such as garlic or onion, is the ideal blood and lymph purifier. To order check high quality health food stores or call 1-800-243-5242.

Chapter 5

The Hormonal Connection

The hormonal link to high blood pressure is vast. Hormones control the majority of bodily processes, including circulation. The pumping power of the heart, as well as the arterial tone, are largely controlled by the hormones.

Why are the hormones so important? It would appear that the heart muscle and the arteries should take precedence. In fact, the heart is merely a muscle and the arteries are merely tubes. Their function is under strict glandular control. What's more, it is the disruption of glandular function that is at issue. This is because when this system is dysfunctional, blood pressure disorders develop.

The heart rate, its pumping power, and its nerve function are directly affected by the glands. So is blood pressure.

The glandular system is readily damaged by stress. If the stress is severe, this system may be neutralized. This usually occurs only as a result of extreme prolonged stress. When this happens, the glands, which are responsible for the maintenance of normal circulation, that is the thyroid and adrenals, become incompetent. Thus, the blood pressure fluctuates, and normal control is lost.

The glands which are primarily involved in blood pressure regulation are the thyroid, adrenals, and pituitary. The testes and ovaries may play a lesser role. Disorders of any such glands may result in blood pressure, as well as heart, disease.

All glands have a considerable reserve for their key functions. The damage must be extensive, that is for them to lose their controls. Severe psychic stress can cause this—the agitation must be prolonged and devastating. So can infection and toxicity. Heavy metals may poison the glands, particularly lead and cadmium. This may readily result in hypertension. The key is to regain normal glandular function.

This is far more important than the intake of any drugs, diuretics, or antagonists. Again, by discovering and treating the cause the condition may be reversed. The major glands which control circulation are the adrenals and the thyroid and to a lesser degree the pituitary. These organs strictly control blood pressure levels. There must be rather severe disease of these organs in order for the blood pressure mechanism to falter. The fact is persistent high blood pressure is evidence of disease in these organs. The disease could be due to toxicity, nerve damage, nutritional deficiency, and/or infection, the latter being the primary factor.

Stress greatly damages the endocrine glands. This is why stress may lead to high blood pressure.

Adrenal disorders: the missing link?

Medical textbooks seemingly neglect the role of adrenal dysfunction as a cause of high blood pressure. Even so, there is mention of specific diseases of the adrenals, that is hypersecretion of these glands, as a potential cause. The latter is known as Cushing's Syndrome. Here, the adrenal glands produce an excess of hormones, which leads to fluid retention and, therefore, high blood pressure. This excess of hormones may be due to either infection or adrenal tumors, perhaps stress. Here, the adrenals over-produce a certain hormone, aldosterone, resulting in fluid and salt retention. This increase in salt, and, thus, water, increases blood volume, which forces the heart to work harder. The arteries become stretched, that is due to the massive increase in fluid volume. As a result, the blood pressure increases. Yet, there is a revelation as a result of this disease: could all cases of hypertension have an adrenal component? Could this disease be, in fact, a kind of adrenal exhaustion? However, it is what damages the adrenal glands that is of concern, not, for instance, salt per se. In other words salt—sodium chloride—by itself rarely, if ever, causes high blood pressure.

It is well known that stress aggravates and/or causes high blood pressure. It is the adrenal glands which bear the brunt of this damage. Prolonged psychic stress greatly damages them. Yet, the most toxic form of stress that influences these glands, that is in terms of high blood pressure, is anger. Rage and anger are the major emotional factors in high blood pressure. Depression and apathy also play a role. Yet, it is hostility which is the most damaging. If the anger and/or rage is continuous, ultimately, high blood pressure, as well as heart disease, develops. A peaceful heart— a heart and soul which are at ease—in such an individual high blood pressure rarely if ever develops. Thus, in this disease there is virtually always an emotional factor.

Anyone can be at ease. The best way is to trust, that is in a higher purpose: the authority of almighty God. This is an invaluable arena, that is to broach the issue of an individual's internal feelings—his or her faith. This is no attempt to preach: it is simply a scientific fact. Modern research proves that people who have some form of belief—some kind of belief in an almighty power—are far less vulnerable to disease than people who fail to believe. In fact, people who trust in a higher power are far less vulnerable to the development of mental disorders than their non-believing brethren. Thus, trusting only helps the individual, providing peace in a chaotic world.

There are great benefits in trusting in a person's purpose; that is in the fact that each person belongs to an almighty Lord. What's more, it makes sense to trust. People had to arise from a Source. Each human being is different. The brain is highly sophisticated, as is the body. In other words, the human being is utterly unique. Such a being could only be the result of a plan. This means that there must also be a Planner. People who believe in such a purposeful existence, that life itself has a critical meaning, are at relative peace, which is manifested in improved health. Anger, jealousy, hate, and agitation, as well as disbelief, can only result from a sick heart. By having, rather, creating, peace in the heart the individual can ease his/her burdens. This will add years to life and diminish the risks for the development of high blood pressure, heart disease, arthritis, cancer, and other serious diseases.

For high blood pressure to develop there is often a lack of peace. If a person is constantly thinking about what he/she fails to have or what the next person has, this will result in mental chaos. The stress from this alone is enough to kill an individual. Here, if a person realizes that all will eventually end—that is the nature of things—and that all begins with God and, what's more, all will return to Him, the fact is this will allow the person to be at peace. As a result, the heart will be eased.

Anger and jealousy, as well as self pity, are the evils of the human race. They are evil, because they destroy the individual, preventing his or her success. Through anger and jealousy toxic chemicals are produced in the body, which damage the organs, particularly the adrenals. The fact is the adrenal glands bear the brunt of any emotional strain. To be healthy it is crucial to rid the self of such emotional contaminants. Thus, it is important to be at peace truly within. Feelings of hate, anger, and jealousy, as well as self pity, must be eliminated. These are all curses, if a person only knew it. Only then can a person find peace. Only then can voluminous success be gained. As first described by Judy Kay Gray, M.S., self pity is the doom of the individual, fully preventing any forward movement.

To pity the self is to incur the wrath of God. Truly, He hates such thinking, because people who pity themselves are the greatest failures of all. Again, to quote Gray, author of *The Greatest Treasure of All,* "Self pity is the single most destructive of all human emotions." For a person who desires true peace this booklet is highly recommended. This is a highly inspiring book. It is also available as a book and tape kit. It may be read repeatedly. To order *The Greatest Treasure of All* (only available mail-order) call 1-800-243-5242.

Sadly, people are comfortable existing in certain mental zones, including the zone of self pity. Here they exist, preoccupied in their own misery, unhappy and unwilling to change and/or to improve their lives. They are comfortable feeling sorry for themselves. What's more, they relish in engaging others, that is enticing others, to also feel sorry for them. They live here—in this zone—because they are used to it. To attempt to bring them out of it is a major endeavor, as if pulling a fighting fish from water. They fester in their sick, tired, unhappy, and disenchanted lives, as if to say, "Life has been unfair to me." As a result, they only deepen their misery, feeding their hearts and souls with negative impressions. They retain their anger, fuming and festering, with no outlet. Such individuals are prime candidates for high blood pressure.

There are numerous disorders of the glands, which may result in high blood pressure as well as cardiovascular disease. Cushing's syndrome is an excellent model of the role of the adrenals in blood pressure disorders. By studying this disorder the appropriate cures can be discerned. This syndrome is due to a kind of hyperactivity of these glands, usually due to gross pathology, although severe stress can precipitate it. The direct cause of the high blood pressure is the increase in blood levels of a group of steroids, known as the glucocorticoids, again, the latter being produced by the adrenals. The more common name for these steroids is cortisol.

This condition was first discovered in the 1930s by, appropriately, Harvey Cushing, M.D. It is characterized by a thickening of the body, known as truncal obesity, as well as exhaustion, weakness, lack of menstruation, male-pattern hair growth (in women), swelling, stretch marks on the abdomen and buttocks, edema, thinning of the bones and easy fractures. In the extreme, it can result in glucose in the urine, and, ultimately, diabetes. The condition is usually caused by excess cell growth in the adrenals, which may be due to toxic damage to these glands. The source for this excessive cell growth may arise in a distant organ: the pituitary. A tumor in the latter may agitate the adrenals, causing excessive cell growth. More rarely, it is due to a primary tumor of the adrenals or chronic infection, that is tuberculosis.

Chronic infection appears to be the major factor in this disease. Recent evidence indicates a toxin is produced in the body, which destroys the adrenals. Somewhere in the body there is a site of infection, which is poisoning these glands, leading to excessive cell growth and/or tumors. Potential sites of the chronic infection include the teeth, gums, sinuses, lungs, and intestines. Infections and/or disease of the thyroid, including thyroid tumors and cancer, may also play a role.

It makes sense that in order to reverse high blood pressure the adrenal glands must be bolstered. What's more, any site of chronic infection, which damages these glands, must be eradicated.

Boosting the function of these glands is critical. The adrenal glands are readily exhausted. When this occurs, they become vulnerable to infection. These glands have a high need for vitamin C. When this vitamin is lacking, the adrenals are readily attacked. Thus, it is crucial to keep them regularly supplied with significant amounts of vitamin C.

Natural-source vitamin C effectively supports the adrenals. To strengthen these glands take Purely-C, three capsules twice daily. This may also be taken sublingually, that is Purely-C drops, five to ten drops three times daily. Also, increase the consumption of vitamin C-rich foods, including kiwi, papaya, oranges, grapefruit, lemons, limes, tangerines, strawberries, broccoli, and spinach (raw). However, do not eat an excess of vegetables. The adrenal glands thrive on salty foods, particularly animal foods. Avoid substances which destroy vitamin C, notably cigarette smoke, alcohol, solvents, sulfites, and aspirin. Regarding the latter a single pill can destroy 20 milligrams of vitamin C. Thus, daily aspirin intake rapidly creates the deficiency. Sugar also destroys the vitamin, that is it oxidizes it.

Royal jelly is another invaluable aid. It directly nourishes the glands. A high grade undiluted form of royal jelly is available. This royal jelly is fortified with special herbs, which boost, and, in fact, normalize adrenal function. Known as Royal Power, it naturally boosts adrenal function.

The regular intake of Royal Power, as well as crude natural vitamin C, helps normalize adrenal function, which is crucial for reversing hypertension. Remember, stress is a major cause of hypertension, and this is because it causes great damage to the adrenal glands. What's more, stress causes the loss of vitamin C, creating a vicious cycle. Thus, the combination therapy, Purely-C plus Royal Power, helps reverse the very causes of stress-induced hypertension. The fact is vitamin C greatly strengthens natural adrenal function. This combination therapy is the natural way to normalize adrenal capacity.

Any hidden infections must also be destroyed. This can be achieved through the intake of spice oil extracts, that is the Oreganol and CardioClenz. What's more, for deep-seated adrenal glandular or tissue infections, such as deeply rooted systemic candidiasis or tubercular adrenal glandular infection, the OregaBiotic multiple spice capsules may be necessary, three capsules twice daily. For people with sensitive systems the Oregabiotic must be taken with a full meal. What's more, to increase its efficiency take it with a shot glass of extra virgin olive oil. The wild oregano/spice extracts will help eradicate noxious pathogens, which may be deeply rooted within the glands as well as other tissues such as the sinuses, tonsils, and gums.

Is salt poisonous?

Medical textbooks claim that salt restriction is the primary therapy for hypertension. True, restricting salt lowers blood pressure. It does so but by a bizarre mechanism: volume depletion. In other words, by forcibly lowering the salt the body also loses blood volume. Yet, the body needs blood volume to maintain blood flow to critical organs, including the brain and the heart itself. Salt is the main electrolyte in the blood, needed to specifically hold fluid in the blood vessels. Thus, salt restriction interferes with the very purpose for which it was designed, the prevention of circulatory catastrophes. The real purpose of salt restriction is artificial: to gain a temporary reduction in blood pressure. This amounts to merely treating the symptoms, because the fact is salt by itself is far from the cause of high blood pressure. What's more, salt restriction has another ominous result: adrenal gland damage. These glands are dependent upon salt. This is because the adrenal glands produce a critical hormone needed to maintain circulatory balance: aldosterone.

The very purpose of this hormone is to prevent salt loss. It is salt which is needed to maintain blood volume. It is the blood volume which keeps the heart pumping and the blood flowing to the critical organs. Eventually, due to forcible salt restriction the ability of the adrenal glands to produce this critical hormone is compromised. Ultimately, the glands become exhausted, even damaged. In the extreme the damage becomes life-threatening, leading to a condition known as Addison's disease. The latter can be readily caused by salt restriction. Thus, the medical therapy for high blood pressure, severe salt restriction, causes a greater degree of damage than any benefit.

It is well known that anti-hypertensive drugs deplete salt. The fact is this is the purpose of many of these drugs. Many anti-hypertensive drugs are diuretics, which means they cause water loss. Again, when water is lost, so are nutrients, including sodium and chloride. Yes, salt is a nutrient. The body requires it. Forcing its loss is unhealthy, rather, diabolical. This is because the very existence of the human is dependent upon this substance. Without salt, death will rapidly ensue. The fact is salt loss is a major cause of sudden death, particularly in heart disease patients. Congestive heart failure may well be a salt deficiency syndrome, as is sudden cardiac collapse, that is heart attack. The regular intake of sea salt, combined with proper adrenal support, that is the Royal Power, will largely prevent heart attacks.

Heart rhythm disturbances, as well as mitral valve prolapse, may also be caused primarily by salt deficiency. The heart is fully dependent upon salts, which are needed for the creation of certain gradients within the heart muscle cells. These gradients create the basis for the electrical activity of the heart's muscle fibers. Without salt heart function is fully compromised.

Salt, that is natural unprocessed salt, is no poison. It is a necessary part of a person's diet. It is virtually impossible to live without it. Salt restrictive diets only create additional health problems. There is no long-term benefit from such diets: only ultimate loss, not only in health and the risk for premature death but also in the enjoyment of food and life. The risks for heart attacks are far higher in people who strictly avoid salt than in salt consumers. Incredibly, the avoidance of salt fails to decrease the risks for heart disorders.

Sea salt: the safe alternative

The body requires salt. Without it death rapidly ensues. It is a critical nutrient. A deficiency of salt, that is a lack of sodium and chloride, results in a wide range of symptoms. These symptoms include dizziness, palpitations, confusion, irritability, exhaustion, muscle fatigue, muscle cramps, nervousness, insomnia, and dozens of others. The fact is many high blood pressure patients, especially those on diuretic drugs or who are following a low sodium diet, can relate to these symptoms. Adding salt to the diet quickly eliminates them. Incredibly, the moderate intake of sea salt, especially the crude unprocessed kind, may help lower blood pressure. In contrast, severe salt restriction may lead to a rise in blood pressure. This is a reverse reaction, in fact, a compensation for the loss of this critical element.

Low sodium levels are common, especially in people under medical care for high blood pressure or other forms of heart disease. It is dangerous to have a low sodium status. The body requires this substance, that is to maintain blood flow. Excessively low sodium levels can even lead to death, that is through heart collapse, heart failure, heart attack, and even stroke. It was Alderman, of New York's Cornell University

College of Medicine, who thoroughly proved this. He noticed that men with low blood levels of sodium readily died from heart attacks. When he corrected this sodium and chloride deficiency by giving IV salt solutions, he halted the deaths. Incredibly, as a result of Alderman's therapy the death rate from heart attacks was reduced by some 400%. This is a clear sign that salt is absolutely necessary for the circulatory system and that in the vast majority of cases restricting this substance causes great damage, without benefit. Thus, incredibly, sudden death from heart attack may have more to do with sodium deficiency than a deficiency of any other substance. To live a long and vital life it is necessary to include plenty of natural salt in the diet. Never go on a severe low salt diet.

Alderman's work is mind-boggling, although I long before condemned the low salt diet in *How to Eat Right and Live Longer* as well as in *Nutrition Tests for Better Health.* In fact, I discovered through working with patients the Sodium Wasting Syndrome. In this condition patients are unable to retain sodium, so it must be constantly replaced in the diet, often quite vigorously. Patients are instructed to use as much salt to taste as desired and to purposely eat healthy salty snacks such as salted roasted nuts, salty cheese, salty rice or whole grain crackers, and boiled egg with salt. In addition, in extreme cases salt capsules are consumed. These are made by the patient by filling size two capsules with sea salt and taking one or more with each meal.

Publishing in the prominent journal, *Hypertension,* Alderman made it clear that rather than offering protection low salt diets increase the risk for sudden death, especially from heart attacks. The sodium status was measured in the urine. People with a low urinary sodium level had high levels of a potentially toxic compound: renin. This is evidence of the body's desperate attempt to compensate for the low sodium intake. Yet, it was unable to do so. After following patients for some 4 years it was determined that in particular men with a low urinary sodium level had more than a four-fold increase in heart attacks than those with high sodium levels.

As mentioned previously there is a kind of salt wasting syndrome, which is potentially serious. Here, the body is unable to retain salt, largely due to a defect in adrenal function. Millions of Americans suffer from weakened adrenal glands. This syndrome may be manifested by a wide range of symptoms and conditions. It may be regarded as the great mimicker, and its manifestations are frequently misdiagnosed as vague illnesses, including chronic fatigue syndrome, fibromyalgia, panic attacks, obsessive compulsive syndrome, hypoglycemia, and numerous other conditions. The majority of these conditions are associated with salt depletion. Yet, unfortunately, physicians are largely unaware of it. This is reminiscent of a heart-breaking case: that of a two-year-old child, who craved salt. The child's cravings were extreme. This was a persistent problem seemingly for the parents; they thought the cravings of their daughter were abnormal. Once, they found her on the countertop, attempting to remove the salt from the cupboard. They took her to the doctor, and, incredibly, salt was severely restricted. No attempt was made to determine the reason for the salt cravings. The parents blocked the child from attempting to get salty snacks. As a result, within days the child died. This child suffered from a salt wasting syndrome. The cure would have been to give her large amounts of salt in the form of sea salt and healthy salty snacks. Adrenal support, for instance, in the form of the Royal Oil, would also have been curative. The child sought the cure. The doctor and parents denied it. As a result, she died.

Doctors frequently miss the signs and symptoms of sodium/chloride deficiency—to the patient's detriment. Since there is no simple blood test to prove it a self-test has been devised. Now, a person can determine the degree of sodium and chloride deficiency, if any, that they suffer. This fast is derived from the book *Nutrition Tests for Better Health.*

Answer the following questions and add up the score. Unless listed otherwise each question is worth one point. Which of these apply to you?

1. dizziness
2. palpitations
3. confusion
4. irritability
5. insomnia
6. nervousness
7. muscle fatigue
8. muscle cramps or muscle stiffness
9. exhaustion
10. hallucinations
11. lack of appetite
12. cold weather causes urge to urinate
13. frequent urination with small volume
14. diarrhea
15. coldness of extremities
16. paranoia
17. panic sensations
18. low blood pressure
19. nausea/vomiting
20. lack of thirst
21. difficulty concentrating
22. Is your blood cholesterol level particularly low?
23. Do you drink distilled water or reverse osmosis water on a daily basis?
24. Do you drink large quantities of water, that is more than 8 glasses daily?

25. Do you exercise vigorously several times per week?
26. Do you abhor the thought of eating meat?
27. Do you rarely if ever eat red meat?
28. Are you on a low salt diet?
29. Have you severely restricted salt from your diet (add 3 points for this)?
30. Are you unusually sensitive to hot weather, hot showers, etc.?
31. Have you been diagnosed with a low blood sodium?
32. Do you take a diuretic drug on a daily or weekly basis?
33. Do you take several anti-hypertensive drugs on a daily basis (add 3 points for this)?
34. Do you take an anti-hypertensive drug, which specifically depletes sodium (add 4 points for this)?
35. Are you a vegetarian?
36. Are you a strict vegan (add 3 points for this)?
37. Do you have a history of adrenal weakness (Addison's disease or adrenal insufficiency—add 3 points for this)?
38. Do you eat mostly vegetables and little meats?
39. Do you regularly take laxatives?
40. Do you rarely eat salty snacks?
41. Are you under an extreme amount of stress?

Your Score_____

1 to 5 points: Mild sodium deficiency—at this level of deficiency all that is usually needed is to add salt to the diet. Use an unrefined sea salt, about a teaspoon daily. Also, eat salt-rich foods such as organically-raised meats, poultry, and wild fish. In terms of vegetables zucchini is high in sodium.

6 to 12 points: Moderate sodium deficiency—with this score sodium in the form of natural sea salt must be added in the diet immediately. Use salt heavily on all foods. Eat healthy salty

snacks such as natural pickles, olives in brine, salted roast organic beef, turkey, or chicken, boiled egg with salt, and salted nuts. Eat plain full fat yogurt and add plenty of salt. Eat a salty snack between meals. What's more, to strengthen the adrenal glands take a high potency undiluted royal jelly product, that is the Royal Power, 4 capsules every morning. Commercial royal jelly products, that is the royal jelly capsules, are diluted. The Royal Power is full strength. Also, take the sublingual form, the Royal Oil, a half teaspoon once or twice daily. Avoid the intake of refined sugar, since it damages the adrenal glands and disturbs salt balance.

13 to 19 points: Severe sodium deficiency—This is a danger zone. Correct the sodium loss/deficiency immediately by taking in the diet 2 to 3 teaspoons of crude sea salt daily. Also, eat salty snacks between meals. Take Royal Power, 6 capsules every morning with breakfast. Also use the Royal Oil, one half teaspoonful twice daily. Avoid the intake of aggressive diuretics such as alcohol, beer, and caffeine. Also, strictly avoid the intake of artificial sweeteners. See your doctor about eliminating any sodium-wasting drugs. Immediately, go off the low salt diet and liberally salt all foods. Strictly avoid refined sugar. It greatly disturbs salt balance.

20 to 28: Extreme sodium deficiency—this is a super-danger zone. Include on the foods and in the diet 4 teaspoons of crude sea salt daily. Regularly snack on salty snacks. Take Royal Power, 4 capsules at breakfast and another 4 at noon. Also, for a direct sublingual effect take the Royal Oil, a teaspoonful twice daily. Have your blood sodium and chloride assessed. If it is low, get routine tests until it is normalized. Avoid the intake of aggressive diuretics such as alcohol, beer, and caffeine. Also, strictly avoid the intake of artificial sweeteners. See your doctor

about eliminating any sodium-wasting drugs. Healthy salty snacks, which can help replenish falling sodium levels, include salted roasted nuts, salted sunflower seeds, salt-coated pumpkin/squash seeds, pickles, olives in brine, feta cheese, salted organic roast beef, chicken, turkey, and sardines. What's more, use a heavy hand with the salt shaker on all foods, particularly vegetables, meats, and potatoes. Strictly avoid refined sugar. It greatly disturbs salt balance.

29 and above: Profoundly extreme sodium deficiency—this is a death zone. Immediately begin using unprocessed sea salt in the diet, as much as desired. What's more, fill several large gelatin capsules with the salt: take two capsules with each meal. Snack on salty snacks, as much as is desired. What's more, the function of the adrenal glands must be boosted. Take Royal Power, four capsules or more three times daily. When symptoms have dissipated, reduce the dose to four to six capsules every morning. Also, for a direct sublingual effect take the Royal Oil, a teaspoonful three times daily.

Strictly avoid the consumption of refined sugar, since it destabilizes the adrenal glands. What's more, avoid all sources of artificial sweeteners. Aspartame poisons the adrenal glands, which aggravates the sodium loss. See your doctor about eliminating any sodium-wasting drugs. Healthy salty snacks, which can help replenish falling sodium levels, include salted roasted nuts, salted sunflower seeds, salt-coated pumpkin/squash seeds, pickles, olives in brine, feta cheese, salted macadamia nuts, salted organic roast beef, chicken, turkey, and sardines. What's more, there is a need to use a heavy hand with the salt shaker on all foods, particularly vegetables, meats, and potatoes. The point is simple. Without salt, a person cannot survive. Major medical journals advise against restricting this substance.

Severe salt restriction may even have the reverse effect, causing a rise in blood pressure. This is due to the enormous stress placed by such a diet upon the adrenal glands. In response to the salt restriction these glands over-produce a hormone, aldosterone, which, in fact, causes water retention, therefore raising blood pressure. As always the approach of modern medicine is catastrophic. The medical model is to forcibly reduce blood volume by restricting salt. It is to also force water out of the tissues, that is through diuretics. It is also to block various receptors, for instance, in the kidneys, in order to artificially lower blood pressure. Rarely if ever is the underlying cause discovered or treated. People remain on potent medications for life, and these drugs have serious side effects which may readily cause a severe reaction, even death. Thus, high blood pressure medicines, by interfering with normal physiology, reduce life span, rarely if ever extending it.

Thyroid dysfunction: a key factor

The thyroid gland is appropriately known as the "Master of Metabolism." It plays an integral role in the rate of metabolic reactions. Thyroid hormone directly influences the internal functions of the cells. A low output of thyroid hormone slows the cells down; too high overworks them.

The cells of the heart are influenced by this hormone. So are the cells of the arteries. Regarding the heart thyroid hormone helps create a normal rhythm. Regarding the arteries it helps keep the metabolic activity in high order to prevent the accumulation of fat or clots.

The metabolism of food is also thyroid-dependent. In particular, the rate of the processing of food, that is the conversion of food to energy, is controlled by it. The thyroid gland is the key organ for converting, for instance, sugars and starches to fuel. It is these carbohydrates which are mainly responsible for fat accumulation in the body. Thus, if the thyroid gland is compromised, the food calories will not be burned, and instead, they will accumulate as fat. This is why high blood fat levels are one of the cardinal symptoms of lowered thyroid output. This condition is known as hypothyroidism.

People with hypothyroidism are highly vulnerable to circulatory diseases. It was Broda Barnes, M.D., who first made the connection. He proved that a deficiency in thyroid output led to the accumulation of fat in the arteries, a condition known as atherosclerosis. He also found that as a result of the defect the heart muscle became weak, making sufferers vulnerable to heart attacks. If the thyroid condition was treated, the signs and symptoms disappeared; the heart attack risk was eliminated. What's more, the fat deposits in the arteries were dissipated. If there was no treatment, inevitably, heart and arterial disorders resulted, including high blood pressure and elevated cholesterol.

The thyroid is dependent upon a single mineral for its function: iodine, a component of the seas. This mineral is also found in the Earth but in smaller quantities. From the soil it is readily absorbed into the food; fish become enriched in it by eating smaller creatures and by, in fact, bathing in it.

Seafood truly feeds the thyroid, because it is rich in a type of iodine that is well absorbed by the body. Studies have shown that regular seafood eaters have relatively normal glands, while people who eat mainly meat and other "land-based" foods have slightly enlarged glands. Seafood provides a variety of nutrients required by this gland, including vitamin B_6, niacin, magnesium, iodine, zinc, and the amino acid tyrosine.

In the Western world disorders of the thyroid are epidemic. For instance, some 40 million North Americans suffer from at least some degree of this disorder. This is nearly one in eight people. There are primarily two types of thyroid dysfunctions: hypothyroidism and hyperthyroidism, the former being by far the most common.

In hypothyroidism the first sign is often a sensitivity to cold or perhaps fatigue. Patients may tend to wear extra layers of clothes, even wearing a sweater or socks to bed. There may also be various mental symptoms, including memory loss, depression, confusion, and, particularly, poor concentration. A kind of apathy may develop, and there is an intolerance to exercise. There may be a loss in physical drive, including sexual desire, and the ability to make decisions and carry out plans is compromised. As the disease progresses a physical transformation may occur. The person may become bloated. The skin of the face may become noticeably thick, even doughy. In the extreme the entire face, as well as the neck, may appear swollen. Even the eyelids become puffy. The lips and tongue become thickened, as do the mucous membranes of the throat, nose, and sinuses. This may result in unrelenting snoring as well as mouth breathing.

Due to a thickening of the vocal cords the voice becomes hoarse; the pitch of the voice is often lowered. Despite a rather modest appetite such individuals may rapidly gain weight, while finding weight loss virtually impossible. Headache, which may be severe, often develops. The headaches can be frequent: even daily. Constipation is also common. Exhaustion is routine; the person may even become easily breathless on the most minimal exercise. The menses are irregular; there may even be serious menstrual disorders such as endometriosis and uterine fibroids.

The heart is adversely affected. According to Hoskins in his book, *Endocrinology*, the slow metabolic state causes a kind of malnutrition of the heart, making it weak. What's more, in this condition the metabolism within the arteries themselves is slowed. Thus, the arteries are unable to process and burn fat. This leads to the accumulation of fat, as well as cholesterol, within the arteries. The fact is a moderately high cholesterol level in an individual who is suffering from some degree of tiredness, exhaustion, and weight disturbances is a tell-tale sign of hypothyroidism. Thus, in hypothyroidism all the major risk factors for high blood pressure develop, that is a sluggish heart, poor circulation, thickening of the blood, high cholesterol, high triglycerides, and weakened heart muscle.

All this can be reversed by the appropriate therapy. This includes a diet rich in iodine, including that from animal sources, plus the intake of a high grade iodine/kelp supplement. Thyroset (formerly ThyroKelp) is a formula based upon high-grade natural iodine sources. The primary active ingredient is a special kind of wild kelp found in the far northern oceans. Wild kelp contains the thyroid hormone precursor, diiodotyrosine. This is what makes northern Pacific fish, such as the King Salmon and halibut, so powerful. They thrive among the natural kelp beds; perhaps this accounts for their great strength. Thyroset is the only thyroid-support supplement containing northern Pacific kelp. This is a natural form of iodine combined with wild herbs, as well as the amino acid, tyrosine, which bolster thyroid function. Thyroset may be safely taken with thyroid medication. Incredibly, it helps reduce the need for such medication.

The role of stress: the depletion of hormones

Stress has been directly tied to high blood pressure. Yet, rarely does this alone cause it. Usually, there are underlying causes; stress merely perpetuates it.

Stress depletes adrenal reserve. In fact, it negatively affects all glands. Severe prolonged stress damages the glands, increasing the risks for circulatory diseases. Hans Selye, author of *The Stress of Life,* clearly documented its direct ill effects on the glands. He determined that the entire glandular system was affected by psychological stress as well as physical stress. In his detailed investigations he found that as a result of stress actual physical, as well as chemical, changes occur in organs. The stressful agent, or thought, first affected the brain, then the pituitary and then the rest of the body, including the adrenal glands, thyroid gland, lymph nodes, thymus, and white blood cells. People who fail to allow themselves to be stressed and who rarely if ever entertain negative thoughts have healthier organs than those who think negatively and who succumb to stress.

The excess output of cortisone has a negative affect on the body. It is directly tied in some individuals to a rise in blood pressure. In the natural cures plan the adrenals will be nourished, so that they can heal and so they can respond normally to stress instead of hyper-responding.

In order for the hypertension to be reversed the individual must learn to control his/her stress. Each person has control of his/her own emotions. Here, there is total control: to be either happy or miserable, feel good or poorly, experience love or anger, and to be positive or morose. Each person can decide to either be at peace or disturbed—to feel vital about life or despondent. Anger, hate, jealousy, guilt feelings, remorse, anxiety, and apathy devastate glandular function. Such emotions also devastate the immune system. The solution is to feel good about your circumstances regardless of the issues. It is to have the most upbeat, positive attitude possible—at all times. It is to be of good countenance, that is of good cheer. This will only help the individual, while if he/she succumbs to the negativity of his/her own mind, all that will result is loss.

Here is the best advice possible for keeping the hormonal system in high condition. It is to be consistently as positive as possible. Go out of your way to be vitally positive. Be excessively positive. Allow yourself to be profusely happy. This will help the individual's health more than any other advice. This is how the glands can be quickly healed. What's more, never immerse the self in remorse or guilt sensations. These emotions devastate adrenal glandular function. So, stay super-positive. Plus, take the appropriate nutritional and herbal medicine. This will help the person remain in balance and help prevent stress-induced hormonal disorders. What's more, to naturally balance the thyroid take a potent adrenal supplement, that is the Royal Power, three capsules twice daily and one teaspoon of Royal oil twice daily. You will soon feel the difference.

Chapter 6

Natural Cures

Regarding high blood pressure there is no need to despair. Nature has the answers. The fact is, originally, all high blood pressure remedies were based upon nature: herbs and herbal extracts, with potent pharmaceutical powers. Only later in the mid-twentieth century were they synthesized, that is their active ingredients, into drugs. Yet, this was not for health purposes but, rather, for financial gain. An early medical journal from the 1950s, *Circulation,* proves the point. A number of the drugs recommended for heart and circulatory diseases, including digoxin and rauwolfian alkaloids, are herbal. In one ad the exact source of the drug is described: the root extract of *Rauwolfia serpentina.* Thus, as little as 50 years ago high blood pressure was treated by medical doctors with herbs. Now, suddenly, there is a push to regulate or even restrict herbs. This is never for human safety. Rather, it is for the protection of vested interests. The fact is the major *chemical* cause of death is drugs as well alcohol and tobacco. Such toxins outright kill a half million or more Americans yearly. Again, it is the powers behind such toxins which are attempting to regulate herbs, not any public interest.

Herbal diuretics: the natural answer

Diuretic drugs fail to cure heart disease. In fact, they perpetuate it, largely as a result of their toxic actions upon the kidneys. What's more, such drugs deplete critical nutrients needed for the maintenance of normal blood pressure. Such nutrients include folic acid, thiamine, vitamin B_6, magnesium, potassium, sodium, chloride, and zinc.

Of note both folic acid and vitamin B_6 are required for the metabolism of homocysteine. The latter chemical, if allowed to accumulate, apparently damages the heart and arteries. B_6 and folic acid speed the detoxification of this compound. A deficiency of these vitamins increases the risks for heart disease due to the toxic effects of homocysteine upon the cardiovascular system. To determine the degree of B_6 and folic acid deficiency see Dr. Cass Ingram's *Nutrition Tests for Better Health.* Furthermore, magnesium, which is aggressively destroyed by diuretic drugs, is required for muscle relaxation.

The walls of the arteries are muscular. If magnesium is lacking, the body becomes tense. This is why intravenous magnesium, as well as magnesium supplements, have been found to reduce blood pressure. Zinc is needed to speed healing of damaged tissue, including the lining of the artery walls. In the Western world today zinc deficiency is rampant, especially in people on restrictive diets, including vegans and vegetarians. Potassium is necessary for the activity of the nerves, that is it is the key substance for keeping nerve impulses flowing.

By destroying the aforementioned nutrients drugs interfere with normal metabolism. They disrupt the vital chemistry of the body. Regarding circulatory diseases they create a loss, never any gain. How can a therapy be of value if it damages the very substances which the body needs for normality? It can by no means help. In contrast, herbal and, in fact, food-based, diuretics, help heal, that is regenerate, the body. They enhance the normality, in fact, revive it. They feed the body the minerals it needs, never depleting them. These are the diuretics recommended in this book: the CranFlush and the WildPower Tea. These natural diuretics are made from foods, which are, in fact, wild. Thus, they are more correctly a food rather than a medicine, although their medicinal properties rival any drug.

CranFlush is far superior to the typical cranberry-based supplements. This is because only CranFlush is derived exclusively from wild high bush cranberries, which are far more potent in their diuretic and antiseptic powers than their commercial relatives, as is demonstrated by the following.

CASE HISTORY:

Mrs. M. is a 50-year-old woman with a history of repeated E. coli infections of the bladder. She is naturally oriented and follows a healthy diet, yet, even so, she is plagued with this condition. She had tried a number of herbal compounds and diuretics, with only minimal results. At her next attack I prescribed the CranFlush. She noticed immediate improvement, and within 24 hours the problem was eliminated. What was normally a week of agony was eliminated in only a few hours, all because of the powers of wild cranberry extracts.

Wild cranberry is a potent diuretic. What's more, it is a vigorous antiseptic. Studies show that it contains substances which are highly antibacterial and antifungal. These berries are so powerful in their antibacterial and antifungal activities that while on the bush for months they fail to decay. CranFlush is a dependable cure for any urinary tract infection. What's more, it helps flush from the body excess fluid. Since hypertension is associated with both kidney infection and fluid retention the CranFlush is the preferred cure. What's more, these drops are completely safe and may be used by all age groups. This is the perfect natural cure for children, since it tastes relatively good, readily mixes with juice and is completely non-toxic. What's more, it is highly effective both for bladder and kidney disorders, including acute infections. It is the ideal urinary antiseptic for pets and is particularly ideal for cats with cystitis. Compared to other cranberry extracts the reason it is unique is that it is exclusively made from wild raw unsweetened cranberries. To order CranFlush call 1-800-243-5242 and in Canada, 1-866-377-7423.

Is hypertension a scurvy-like disease?

Vitamin C deficiency is directly related to high blood pressure. While the government 'authorities' are mandating against salt intake, vitamin/mineral status is never mentioned. Consider the tissues, which are diseased in this condition: the gums, teeth, arterial walls, heart valves, veins, and heart muscles. All are highly dependent upon vitamin C. Without this vitamin all such tissues degenerate. What's more, many of the drugs which induce this condition, for instance, cortisone, alcohol, tobacco smoke, and Prednisone, destroy vitamin C.

It is well known that in hypertension there is wholesale degeneration of the arterial walls. What's more, often, the heart valves become diseased, which is manifested by degenerative changes, including scarring. All the components of the circulatory system may be involved: the arteries, veins, heart,

heart valves, and capillaries. All are dependent upon vitamin C. In its absence all degenerates.

Yet, no one should be surprised by these findings. Consider varicose veins. This condition is proven to be related to vitamin C and bioflavonoid deficiency. The same occurs in the arteries, although it is not so obvious, since they are deeper structures and are more resistant to breakdown than the veins. Thus, there may be vitamin C deficiency-induced bleeding, which goes undiagnosed. Even so, certain warning signs of arterial breakdown may develop. Such warning signs include easy bruising, blood vessels, which break under trauma, painful blood blisters, breakouts of tiny red lesions, nose bleeds, bleeding from the kidneys or colon, and hemorrhoids.

Yet, the gums are perhaps the greatest indicators for early vitamin C deficiency. With the lack of this vitamin the tissues become weak. The fact is receding gums is a common condition in individuals diagnosed with hypertension. In many instances people with this disease also suffer from arthritis, that is degeneration of the connective tissue of the joints. All these syndromes are also seen in scurvy. Thus, it is reasonable to place hypertension in the category of nutritional deficiency diseases, notably a deficiency of vitamin C and associated factors. These factors are known as bioflavonoids.

In nature vitamin C and the bioflavonoids always occur together. Today, there is a tendency to take vitamin C by itself, often in megadoses. This violates nature. The bioflavonoids work with the vitamin C for the most desirable effect: the creation of strong vital cells. No such action can be achieved with the synthetic.

Vitamin C and the associated bioflavonoids are required for strengthening blood vessel walls: by itself this vitamin fails to achieve this. Without both these factors the arterial walls, as well as the lining of the heart, degenerate. So do the gums. This may explain the growing proof for the benefits of flavonoid-rich foods, such as red grapes, pomegranates, and sour berries, in the prevention and reversal of this disease. Such fruit are rich in flavonoids, which are required for the optimal utilization of vitamin C. What's more, regular eaters of fresh fruit have a reduced incidence of both arterial disease and high blood pressure, which, again, indicates a critical role for the vitamin. Plus, the regular intake of vitamin C-rich foods and/or natural vitamin C supplements is the best insurance against potentially fatal microbial attack of the circulatory system.

The mechanism of action of these substances is interesting. When vitamin C and/or bioflavonoids are lacking, the tissues of the body, particularly the tissues lining the arteries and heart, become weak. As a result the cells are unable to remain tight against each other. This is because vitamin C is required for the synthesis of cellular glue, the so-called grounding substance. This is descriptive: the cells are 'grounded' when there is plenty of vitamin C and disjoined when it is lacking. Essentially, gaps form between the cells, making them vulnerable to invasion. Normally, with strong cellular glue invasion is impossible. This weakness and the resulting infection is all due to vitamin C deficiency.

Naturally occurring vitamin C, biologically, is different from the synthetic. Only the natural type can be relied upon as a high blood pressure cure. Vitamin C can be consumed both as food and supplements. However, the typical health food store supplements contain primarily synthetic vitamin C. The latter is made from corn, which is largely genetically engineered. This means that the majority of synthetic vitamin C supplements are made from genetically engineered components and, thus, must be avoided. Instead, take a completely natural vitamin C supplement such as the Purely-C.

There is a vitamin C supplement available, which is free of synthetic vitamin C. The vitamin C in it comes exclusively from fruit and herbs. It is available both in capsules and a liquid form. Each tablespoon contains 40 mg of naturally occurring vitamin C, while each capsule contains nearly 60 mg. This is the Purely-C (formerly known as Flavin-C) all natural vitamin C capsules and sublingual drops. The vitamin C in these products is from the tropical fruit, acerola cherries and camu camu, along with rose hips and the sour Mediterranean berry, *Rhus coriaria.* Some people prefer to take both supplements, the drops in juice, in smoothies, or under the tongue, and the capsules as a regular convenient dose. Both are non-irritating for people with sensitive stomachs and are safe, even for infants. These supplements may also be safely given to pets. The regular intake of naturally occurring vitamin C will keep the arteries strong and prevent arterial degeneration. What's more, the gums will become stronger, which will also ward off disease. Remember, healthy, that is strong, gums are a primary defense against heart disease. In this regard, the regular intake of naturally occurring vitamin C is essential in the prevention of arterial and heart diseases. In contrast to commercial vitamin C there is nothing genetically engineered in these supplements.

Through diet alone people fail to get sufficient vitamin C. This is especially true of smokers and drinkers. What's more, those who work in a smoky environment readily become deficient. Stress also depletes this vitamin. The typical American diet is far too low in vitamin C, that is to meet the tissue needs demanded by the modern, stressful life. What's more, the fruit today is relatively low in the vitamin, that is compared to the fruit eaten by our ancestors. Fruit is commonly picked unripe and gas-ripened.

It is the sun, which creates the synthesis of vitamin C. Green fruit, for instance, unripe oranges and grapefruit, may contain little or none of the vitamin. It was Michael Colgan, Ph.D., formerly of the Rockefeller Institute, who proved the scope of this debacle. Testing supposedly ripe oranges at various supermarkets, incredibly, he found that certain oranges had no measurable vitamin C. Thus, even for heavy fruit eaters supplements are necessary. Yet, if fruit is a known cure, recall that, originally, scurvy was cured with citrus fruit, why depend upon the synthetic? Any supplemental sources must be exclusively natural, because natural vitamin C has curative powers within the tissues, while the synthetic fails to achieve this.

With natural vitamin C supplements it may be necessary to take significant quantities; for instance, on a daily basis a tablespoon or two of Purely-C liquid and six to eight capsules of the Purely-C (encapsulated form). Once the tissue levels of this vitamin are built up, a minimal or maintenance amount may be taken, for instance, one half the aforementioned amount.

The work of Szent-Gyorgyi edifies the importance of the natural versus the synthetic. Twice a Nobel laureate, Szent-Gyorgyi was instrumental in synthesizing vitamin C. He first isolated it from natural sources, incredibly, the adrenal glands of animals as well as paprika. When the natural extract was given to patients, they were cured. However, when he attempted to duplicate this with the synthetic, it failed, that is no cures were achieved. This is compelling evidence that the divine, that is the natural, formula is unique, in fact, superior to the synthetic. True, such supplements are lower dose; a few milligrams versus hundreds, even thousands, of milligrams for the synthetics. Yet, biologically, the effects are incomparable.

Crude vitamin C, that is vitamin C from natural substances, is a medicinal agent. It works within the body at a biochemical level, greatly assisting cell and organ function. As mentioned previously numerous bleeding disorders, including nose bleeds, urinary bleeding, and hemorrhoids, have been reversed with natural vitamin C. What's more, these were conditions, which failed to respond to treatment with the synthetic. If possible, only vitamin C from natural sources should be consumed. As a result there will be a significant improvement in health. What's more, with the natural extract there are no side effects. It is well tolerated, even by those with sensitive systems. In contrast, there is a degree of toxicity with the synthetic.

Consider a simple fact: the majority of synthetic vitamin C is derived from corn, the latter being genetically engineered. This effectively rules out synthetic vitamin C as an effective or safe supplemental source. This is because genetically engineered corn contains substances, which are toxic to human beings. Thus, reactions to synthetic vitamin C, including bizarre rashes and digestive disturbances, are becoming increasingly common. Why take chances? Only natural vitamin C should be taken internally. To order natural vitamin C supplements, which are free of any corn derivatives and are devoid of genetically engineered components, check high quality health food stores or call 1-800-243-5242. These supplements, the Purely-C capsules and the Purley-C liquid, are free of any synthetic vitamin C and offer vitamin C exclusively from nature. Do not accept cheap imitations.

Minerals: essential to life

Key activators of cellular reactions minerals are essential to life. Without them cellular function would cease. A critical component of enzymes minerals act as spark plugs, that is without them no activation can occur. The activation is within the cells in the form of enzyme reactions.

Hypertension is associated with mineral deficiencies. These deficiencies may not be the only cause of this condition. However, they play a considerable role. What's more, incredibly, while a sufficient supply of minerals is necessary for the maintenance of normal blood pressure the typical anti-hypertensive drugs greatly deplete them. Common drugs, such as thiazide diuretics and angiotensin blockers, cause magnesium, as well as potassium, deficiency. Certain drugs specifically deplete sodium and chloride. Other minerals which are destroyed by drug therapy include zinc, selenium, and calcium. When evaluating people, it is easy to determine those taking anti-hypertensive medications. All that has to be done is to look at the nails. Invariably, the tell-tale signs will be evident: severe ridges, splitting, peeling, and white spots, all of which are classical signals of mineral deficiency.

Chromium is also critical to arterial health. This may largely be a consequence of its role in blood sugar, as well as fat, regulation. Chromium is also required for muscle metabolism as well as repair. The heart and arteries are largely muscular tissues. The majority of Americans are deficient in this nutrient, which is only found in significant amounts in crude whole grains, blackstrap molasses, various meats, eggs, grape skins, and spices.

Powdered red sour grape is another top source, that is the Resvital powder or capsules. Incredibly, a large heaping teaspoonful contains nearly 50% of the minimal daily requirement of this mineral. That is a massive amount for a natural supplement. This is why Resvital is invaluable for the arteries: it provides natural-source chromium in a form the body can utilize. It is also a top source of naturally occurring potassium. Thus, the Resvital is, essentially, the most unusual of all nutritional supplements, providing a nutrient, which is nearly impossible to procure through common foods. The fact is evidence exists that degeneration of the arteries may be a chromium-deficiency disease.

Enzyme therapy: a key to success

Playing a crucial role in the reversal of high blood pressure, as well as other forms of heart disease, enzymes perform functions no other therapy can match. They are nature's biological machines, capable of performing a host of mechanical and chemical functions. It is the enzymes which spur the digestion of food. It is also these substances which are responsible for stimulating all chemical reactions, for instance, the reactions within the eyes, which process light and the reactions within the nerves that allow feeling. Enzymes control virtually every biological process within the body.

The enzymes also control blood clotting. Blood is incapable of clotting, unless there are sufficient enzymes, to speed the reaction. What's more, these substances help prevent excessive blood clotting. In other words, they help prevent the blood from becoming abnormally thick. This is why they are invaluable for people with high blood pressure.

Enzymes have a kind of living power of their own. They are vital essential molecules, exerting powerful actions, both within cells and in the bloodstream. Even when extracted from the body they exert life-like actions. Not just any enzymes can be relied upon. Only the fruit-based types offer the needed power as well as safety. What's more, the fruit enzymes are vegetarian in source, that is they are completely free of animal by-products. The most potent of these are bromelain and papain. These are also highly safe and have been used in the food industry for years. The pharmaceutical-grade forms of these enzymes, that is the ingredients of Infla-eez, are particularly potent, capable of digesting obstructions, such as the clots and plaques, leading to hypertension. Not every product can achieve these results.

The dissolution of clots and other obstructions is critical for the maintenance of health. The clots become fixed in the arteries, causing damage, swelling, and scarring. This leads to the hard plaques known as atheromas. This causes pressure against the heart, which must pump against them. Infla-eez rapidly dissolves clots as well as obstructions. The enzymes in

Infla-eez are even capable of dissolving germ tissue. The fact is bromelain and papain are nature's chemical roto-rooters. Infla-eez is a combination of pharmaceutical-grade bromelain and papain: a potent combination. The Infla-eez is available in easy-to-digest capsules, made for quick delivery. Studies prove that such enzymes should never be enteric coated, which interferes with their biological activity. These enzymes are active as soon as they are swallowed. This is the most potent vegetable-based enzyme available.

CASE HISTORY:

Mr. C. is a 50-year-old native American, who smokes and is overweight. Playfully, but aggressively, he was wrestling with one of his lodge brothers. He injured his leg, which later became extremely swollen. The pain was severe, radiating to the ankle. Doctors erroneously diagnosed it as an achilles tendon rupture and placed a cast on the leg. The swelling worsened, and a new evaluation proved the cause: a deep blood clot. I saw Mr. C. months after the event and immediately recommended the Infla-eez, along with the Resvital powder and the Oreganol (SuperStrength) rubbed topically all over the leg. Within a month his leg returned to normal, never to bother him again. This was proof of the effectiveness of fruit-source enzymes in dissolving obstructions.

Infla-eez is highly effective against hypertension, especially when combined with the crude red grape powder, that is the Resvital. This is because hypertension is a kind of malignancy of the cardiovascular system, and this is particularly true of severe hypertension. In such cases the arterial walls become enlarged, that is the inside of these walls, due to swellings, resemble tumors. These have a tumor-like name, that is *atheromas*. Infla-eez reverses such swellings. It possesses a kind of anti-tumor action. What's more, its components, high potency bromelain and papain, have been shown to disintegrate fibrin, which is the protein that keeps clots glued together as well as tumors. Fibrin coats various tumors, clots, and swellings, creating a difficult-to-penetrate outer lining. The white blood cells, whose role is to clear all foreign components from the tissues, have a hard time breaking down the fibrin coat. In severe hypertension the heart is forced to work excessively hard, because it pumps against the clots and tumors. This may explain why the bromelain/papain combination is effective against high blood pressure. This is because by dissolving the fibrin coat it helps eliminate arterial obstructions. In the late 1800s British physicians found that extracts from immature papayas, rich in papain, dissolved tumors. More recent research documents how such extracts inhibit the growth of human breast cancer cells.

It is well known that enzyme-rich fruit, such as papaya, star fruit, kiwi, and raw pineapple, aid digestion. This is due to their high content of digestive enzymes. If digestion fails, all organ systems suffer. Harald W. Tietze, author of *Papaya: the Medicine Tree*, notes that through its ability to normalize digestion papaya aids a wide range of diseases, including arthritis, diabetes, and hypertension. The Infla-eez dramatically improves digestion, even cleansing the digestive tract of poisons, harmful germs, and wastes. Regular use greatly improves the digestion and absorption of nutrients, while helping normalize elimination.

The regular intake of enzyme-rich fruit is also beneficial, both for general health as well as in the cure of high blood pressure. The two-week eating plan in Chapter 9 includes plenty of such fruit. There are also recipes for the use of papaya, kiwi, and pineapple. Yet, for a guaranteed potent effect on a daily basis the Infla-eez is invaluable. What's more, due to the high potency of this supplement a higher level effect is achieved than from eating only the fruit. Yet, the combination, that is eating plenty of enzyme-rich fruit, along with the intake of the supplement, is ideal. It was Hippocrates who said, "Death begins in the colon." The fruit-based enzymes are an effective way to stall digestive toxicity by cleansing poisons out of the system in a gentle non-toxic manner. This, combined with the green and/or berry drops, that is the cell cleansing Flush system, purges the colon, as well as the internal cells, of toxins. It is such a purge, which is necessary for ideal health.

When taking Infla-eez along with the intake of enzyme-rich fruit, such as papaya, kiwi, star fruit, wild berries, and raw pineapple, usually, no other digestive enzymes are needed. Bromelain and papain are exceptionally powerful and replace the need for other enzyme supplements. What's more, they are a safer source for supplements than animal-based enzymes, which are largely derived from feedlot cattle and pigs. The latter readily carry germs, which may lead to infection within the body.

CASE HISTORY;

Ms. R., a frail 90-pound 34 year-old woman, was incapable of gaining weight, plus she was plagued with constant digestive symptoms. She was also totally exhausted. Pancreatic enzymes from a well-known maker were prescribed. A week later the patient gave her report: she suffered from agonizing abdominal pain, a severe burning sensation, every time she took the enzymes. What's more, she was left with a constant vague discomfort of the stomach. The enzymes were halted. These pork-based enzymes had apparently infected Ms. R.'s stomach, causing significant discomfort. The manufacturer refused to acknowledge the possibility, claiming their product was germ-free. However, they refused to confirm their claim in writing.

Even though it is potent the Infla-eez cannot damage the stomach or intestines. Rather it greatly aids their functions. It does so by stimulating the digestive process, plus it helps cleanse the gut of toxins and dead cells. Fruit enzymes are excellent cleansing agents for removing various obstructions and contaminants. Thus, not only do they cleanse the arteries but they also remove blockages from the intestines, the colon, and the internal organs.

It has been long believed that since enzymes are proteins they will be inactivated by stomach acid. Thus, according to this belief enzyme pills must be enteric coated, that is with a tough membrane, so they cannot be broken down in the stomach. Yet, research has shown that such coated enzymes are far less potent than the uncoated type, for instance, Infla-eez, which is in mere easy-to-dissolve vegetable gelatin capsules. This makes sense. When a person eats a kiwi fruit, piece of papaya, or pineapple, there is no coating. Why deviate from nature, that is by creating a coating over the enzyme? Research proves the wisdom. Regarding these fruit enzymes they are active in a range of pH: even in the hostile environment of the stomach. Thus, stomach acid fails to inactivate these tough enzymes. What's more, the enzymes are immediately absorbed. Thus, enteric coating stalls their absorption, in fact, prevents it. Avoid enterically coated enzymes. Instead, buy enzyme supplements preferably as capsules, which easily dissolve.

Bromelain-papain-based enzyme supplements, such as Infla-eez, as well as enzyme-rich fruit, have a wide variety of uses. Such plant enzymes are effective in reversing or improving a wide range of diseases, including acne, psoriasis, eczema, vasculitis, arthritis, hardening of the arteries, hypertension, constipation, gout, weak immunity, diabetes, blood clots, fibromyalgia, lupus, scleroderma, and even cancer.

It is the blood clot-dissolving power of such enzymes, which is so invaluable for cancer.

There are several reasons for such an action. Cancer cells spread through the blood, transported on clots. What's more, the tumor surrounds itself with a kind of blood-clot like layer, made from a tough protein known as fibrin. As mentioned previously, fruit enzymes are capable of digesting this layer. Plus, they act as a natural blood thinner, which prevents stickiness of the blood. Sticky blood enhances the spread of cancer cells.

Infla-eez is crucial for the arterial cleansing program. This is because for the full benefits of this therapy to be achieved the hidden clots must be eradicated. This is the purpose of Infla-eez: to bore out all clots, plugs, and obstructions. It is also to help keep the arteries clean, that is to prevent further plugging. This will greatly aid in the prevention of coronary artery disease and, therefore, heart attacks as well as strokes. When combined with the regular intake of enzyme-rich fruit, Infla-eez is a major preventive therapy against heart attacks, strokes, and high blood pressure. People will notice the benefits rather quickly, that is improved blood flow plus a reduction in heart-related symptoms such as angina, chest pain, chest pressure, stagnant veins, high blood pressure, and heart rhythm disturbances.

It is important to realize that it may take a prolonged period to achieve the results. The damage within the arteries has developed over a period of many years, in fact, decades. Thus, it will take time to fully cleanse this system. Ideally, the Infla-eez therapy should be taken for at least 90 days and preferably longer, for instance, six months. A minimal dosage is two capsules on an empty stomach three times daily. It is important to take it on an empty stomach, because food consumes its powers. It may also be taken with food as a digestive aid. However, to gain the roto-rooter-like action within the arteries, it must be taken on an empty stomach.

Wild oregano: dental powerhouse

People think of oregano as a food. Yet, for thousands of years societies have regarded it as a medicine rather than a condiment. The fact is extracts of oregano, that is the wild oregano oil and the concentrated wild oregano/spice capsules, are the mainstay of the anti-infection treatment. Wild oregano, especially its oil extract, is a potent germicide, capable of killing the full range of germs. This is precisely what is needed in the mouth: there are untold numbers of species—germs of all types. An antibiotic would be worthless. A general germicide is ideal.

By destroying dental infections oil of oregano creates another benefit, tightening of the gums:

CASE HISTORY:

Ms. M., a 45-year-old with a history of gum disease, had been receiving consistent warnings from her dentist for the need for gum surgery. She was hesitant, instead trying the oil of wild oregano. She brushed with it twice daily. Upon her next visit her dentist found her gums a perfect pink color and free of any obvious disease. Amazed, he inquired what changes she had made. She told him about the oil, which surprised him. "OK", he said. "Keep on using it."

OregaDENT: triple spice formula for dental health

Oil of clove has a prolonged history as an antiseptic. In the United States it is most well known for its beneficial actions against toothache.

Recent research shows that extracts of clove are universal germicides, capable of killing a wide range of bacteria, viruses, fungi, and parasites. The oil of clove is also a valuable digestive aid, largely curbing sour stomach, bloating, and gas. It is included in this plan, because as a topical germicide, it has a pleasant taste, ideal for application on the gums and teeth. Only the oil of clove *buds* can be used internally. It also has extensive application topically for other various disorders, including cold sores, wounds, and burns. This is an active ingredient of the protective formula, OregaDENT.

Beware of counterfeit oils, which are made from the mere leaves, the latter being inedible. The OregaDENT is made from edible spice oils, and in this regard is useful for eradicating internal infections, including infections of the arteries or valves. It is the ideal topical aid for the teeth and gums, because it offers three novel properties: it is a potent germicide, which is pleasant tasting, it is a powerful antioxidant, and it is an effective anesthetic. This explains its traditional use in dentistry, that is for toothache.

OregaDENT is a combination of three spice oils, notably oils of wild oregano, clove buds, and cinnamon. This is for use on gums and teeth. It can also be added on the toothbrush and dental floss. The alternative is to use the oil of oregano and oil of clove buds separately. Regarding the oil of oregano it can be unpleasant. In contrast, the OregaDENT is pleasant tasting.

Hyper-Ten: herbal regulator

Certain herbs and spices strengthen heart and arterial function. Through this they help normalize blood pressure. Hyper-Ten combines potent herbs and spices precisely for this purpose. Originally produced for high blood pressure, incredibly, it is also effective for a wide range of heart and arterial disorders.

Hyper-Ten contains wild hawthorne berries, long known as regeneratives for the heart and arterial systems. It also contains wild strawberry leaves, a gentle but effective diuretic, as well as red sour grape powder, a rich source of resveratrol. Spices in

Hyper-Ten include wild sage and rosemary, both of which strengthen the heart muscle. Such spice extracts are potent antioxidants, and, thus, they stall arterial wall degeneration. In a patient trial Hyper-Ten proved effective in reducing blood pressure. This is without side effects. It was also proven effective in reducing chest pain, a major secondary effect. This may largely be due to its content of the rare wild hawthorn berries. For hundreds of years these berries have been used to support circulatory health. Scientific studies have shown that the regular intake of such berries increases overall circulation, particularly to the extremities. The berries, as well as the leaves, contain a variety of flavonoids, which are potent antioxidants. These antioxidants apparently interact with the heart and arterial wall, gently decreasing blood pressure. Thus, the combination of antioxidant spices, the natural diuretic, wild strawberry leaves, plus the heart-balancing hawthorn berries, is an ideal means to support the health of the circulatory system. For ideal results Hyper-Ten should be taken with the Sesam-E as well the germicidal supplements mentioned previously. Hyper-Ten is available from health food stores as well as health practitioners and herbally-oriented pharmacies.

Chapter 7

The Eating Plan

Food has an enormous impact upon health. Certainly, what a person eats vastly influences the status of the circulatory system. Certain foods damages it while others preserve, in fact, aid it. Toxic or allergic reactions to certain foods are common, and in susceptible individuals this may result in a rise in blood pressure. The fact is food alone may cause high blood pressure crises.

The plan in this book is to adopt as pure a diet as possible. It is a diet free of noxious additives. Processed foods are prohibited. All such foods irritate the heart and arteries. The fact is these foods cause arterial and heart diseases. Thus, by following the diet alone blood pressure will be reduced.

In this diet the most aggressive foods capable of lowering blood pressure are selected. Some of these foods are the opposite of the standard recommendations: for instance, the emphasis on certain fatty foods such as full fat cottage cheese, organic cheeses, red meat, avocados, eggs. and nuts. However, particularly, regarding milk products, eggs, and meat only organic sources are recommended.

For those who must restrict animal foods nuts and seeds should be regularly consumed. These can to a degree replace the need for a high amount of animal foods. A number of studies have shown that the regular intake of certain nuts, in particular the omega-3-rich walnuts, dramatically reduces the risks for the development of cardiovascular diseases. In one study Spanish investigators, reporting in the medical journal *Circulation*, April, 2004, found that adding walnuts to the diet rapidly improved the health of the arteries, while reducing levels of so-called harmful cholesterol. What's more, nut and seed oils must be regularly consumed. The ideal types for cardiovascular health are oils of walnut, hazelnut, black seed, and sesame. For the treatment of essential fatty acid deficiency oil of pumpkinseed is ideal. All such oils are rich in substances which protect the heart and arteries from degenerating, notably the vitamin E complex. These unrefined nut oils are far superior in their protective effects versus mere synthetic or encapsulated vitamin E.

Fatty foods are essential for the blood pressure reduction plan. They should never be eliminated from the diet. Natural fatty foods are not the main cause of high blood pressure or heart attacks. While this is the opposite of the popular belief such foods help lower blood pressure, since, fat is needed as food by the heart and arteries. In contrast, these organs have little need if any for sugar and starch. The fact is the latter readily disrupt the function of these organs, causing irritation, inflammation, and fluid retention. What's more, the kidneys also depend upon fat as a preferred fuel source. Thus, the majority of critical organs prefer it. Huge amounts of saturated fats are unnecessary, however, a total abstinence of naturally occurring saturated fats will prove harmful. This is because the heart muscle requires a certain amount of such saturated fats for normal function.

Again, it was Guyton, America's most famous physiologist, who claimed that up to 90% of the fuel used by the heart is derived from fat, in other words, of all fuel sources the heart prefers it. As fuel it has little need for carbohydrate and/or protein. This is not necessarily vegetable fat: it is also heavy fats, whether animal or vegetable. So, fat is on this diet, in fact, it is a requirement. The fact is the greater the amount of fat in the diet the better will be the results. Of course, this is only true of healthy all-natural fats.

For those who have high blood pressure this is worth a try. For a month or so simply eat primarily naturally fatty foods, while reducing the intake of carbohydrates. Measure the blood pressure. Quickly, the benefits of fat-rich foods will become obvious.

The emphasis is on heavy fats, that is the fats of olives, avocados, nuts, and seeds plus milk fat, the fat of poultry, meat fat, and eggs. What's more, the main cooking oils, which are recommended, are extra virgin olive oil and butter, which are among the heaviest fats known. Other fats which are encouraged are virgin coconut oil, red palm oil, and cold-pressed sesame oil. For non-cooking oil crude fortified pumpkinseed oil, that is the Pumpkinol, is preferred, along with extra virgin olive oil and Sesam-E oil. Cold-pressed walnut oil may also be used. Certainly, where possible the sources must be organic. It will be noticed that light fats, such as light vegetable oil, Canola oil, and flaxseed oil, are not on the diet. Such fats fail to nourish the internal organs, that is they fail to provide them with fuel. What's more, Canola oil is largely genetically engineered. Thus, it must be strictly avoided.

In this diet vegetables and fruit are included, but the emphasis is on low sugar/starch selections, since in most cases of hypertension there is a degree of carbohydrate intolerance. Potatoes, rice, and grains are too starchy. Their consumption leads to a rise in triglycerides and cholesterol. This leads to stickiness of the blood. Thus, such foods are largely avoided, at least during the initial therapy. After 90 days these foods may be re-introduced into the diet.

Certain sweets, which possess medicinal properties, are allowed. These are foods which have a specific positive action against hypertension. These naturally sweet medicines include pure organic grape juice, organic red and green grapes, pomegranate juice, grapefruit and its juice, and pomegranate syrup. Honey of all types, if truly raw and unprocessed, is also allowed. This is because honey exhibits a number of medicinal actions towards the reversal of this disease. Honey helps normalize fluid balance, because it is hygroscopic. This means it is water-drawing, in other words, it attracts water. Thus, it acts as an osmotic agent, helping maintain normal blood volume. The fact is crude unprocessed honey is such a potent medicine that it rarely if ever raises cholesterol and/or triglyceride levels. Incredibly, in certain individuals, because such honeys are potent antioxidants and because they aid digestion, they help lower such levels.

Crude raw honey, that is the truly wild, natural type, is difficult to find. What's more, it is costly. This is the only kind which can be relied upon as a medicine, as is demonstrated by the following:

CASE HISTORY:

Mrs. S., an 80-year-old Italian immigrant, had a persistent problem with fluid retention, caused by chronic congestive heart failure. The fluid backed up into her lungs, causing respiratory distress and exhaustion. Diuretic drugs had failed to correct the problem: there was seemingly no hope. Her son contacted me, and I recommended medicinal honey, in this case, Super-Market Remedies' Wild Oregano Honey. Within a week the fluid balance was restored and her chest congestion was eliminated.

Honeys of this quality are only available by mail order. These are the truly raw, as well as unfiltered, types, where the bees are never fed sugar. Thus, they are truly medicinal honeys. To order these honeys call 1-800-243-5242. A few stores carry them, notably numerous health food stores in Canada and a few stores in Florida. Regarding Florida contact Nutrition World (Port St. Lucie) and Tunies (Coral Springs). In Canada call 1-866-drspice.

The menus have been carefully selected to create the greatest impact: the most powerful anti-hypertensive actions possible. Specific foods which fight hypertension, such as raw pineapple, raw papaya, grapes, radishes, horseradish, oregano, fresh organic yogurt, wild rice, fatty fish, papaya, kiwi fruit, grapefruit, wild berries, wild honey, nuts, and seeds, have been strategically included. It will also be noticed that there is a Mediterranean flair to this plan. This makes sense, since the Mediterranean diet has been associated with a longer life span and a reduced risk for circulatory diseases than the typical Western diet. This approach plus the appropriate supplements provides the individual with the optimal opportunity to reverse this disease, once and for all.

Yet, regardless of any previous conceptions there is no need to fear the fat content of these meals. As quoted earlier medical textbooks make it clear that the organs need fat, even the heart and arteries. Without it, the circulatory organs degenerate. The arterial wall, as well as the heart muscle, is dependent upon fat in the form of fatty acids as fuel. If such fat is restricted, the cells of these organs degenerate.

Remember, the Inuit ate vast quantities of fat and never developed heart disease, that is until adopting the Western diet. Incredibly, sugar, refined starch, white rice, canned food, candy, margarine, deep fried foods, and similar processed foods are what is now killing them. The fact is the synthetic oils, which contaminate metabolism, are one of the most dangerous of all human toxins, since these oils are effectively destroying the health of the modern man as well as the primitive races. This is proven while the natural, that is God-given, fats are utterly harmless. Margarine, hydrogenated oils, and partially hydrogenated oils, which are products of big industry, have caused a greater number of deaths, particularly from cancer, in the primitive populations than any other factor. Thus, this is terrorism in a package.

There is no harm in natural fat, and it does not cause high blood pressure. Fat is used by the body as a fuel. The highly stressed heart needs a certain amount of fat. It burns it as fuel, since fat in the form of fatty acids is over twice as efficient as a fuel source as sugar. Do not deny your heart the fuel it needs by following an excessively strict low fat diet. The fact is by regularly eating natural fats there will be a dramatic result: an obvious and, ultimately, permanent drop in blood pressure. Again, the best way to prevent a heart attack is to consume as the beneficial fats in the most natural forms possible. So, eat and enjoy, without worry.

TWO WEEKS OF EATING RIGHT

*denotes recipe found in recipe section

Day 1

Breakfast
- steak from grass-fed beef or North Star bison steak plus

organic eggs (2 eggs over easy: this keeps the natural vitamin A in the yolk intact)
- Large glass grapefruit juice (fresh squeezed is best; contains vitamin C, folic acid, and potassium)
- Tablespoon cold-pressed crude sesame oil (Sesam-E)

Lunch
- Simple Sardine Salad*
- a few slices of organic cheese
- Mineral water or V-8 juice

Dinner
- Roasted Organic Chicken in Peanut Sauce
- Steamed broccoli (drink any remaining juice; high in vitamin C and potassium)
- Wild rice with minced onions and garlic

Day 2

Breakfast
- Bowl full-fat organic cottage cheese dusted with tablespoon of Nutri-Sense (provides vitamins A and D and protein, plus B vitamins); top with fresh fruit, i.e. papaya, kiwi, and/or strawberries
- One or two pieces of whole grain or sprouted grain bread (coarse type found in health food stores); spread with organic butter and nut butter. Use crude raw honey as a spread

Lunch
- High Blood Pressure-Beating Hamburger*
- Olive Oil-Enriched Spinach and Yogurt Salad*
- Sesame Seed Paste-Plus*

Dinner
- Wild Salmon With Special Vegetables and Hot Mustard*
  (Two droppersful of GreensFlush: helps cleanse mercury
  residue from the teeth and all fish have some mercury)
- Pumpkinol-Dressed Chopped Salad*
- Bowl organic strawberries in heavy cream or whole milk

Day 3

Breakfast
- Mediterranean Omelet*
- Glass fresh-squeezed orange juice
- Oat Bran Cereal*
- Tablespoon cold-pressed Oil of Wild Black Seed

Lunch
- Healthy Wild Salmon Salad*
- Cold Creamy Squash and Onion Soup*

Dinner
- Baked wild halibut (provides immune-building protein and
  fatty acids; the fatty acids are antiinflammatory); bake with
  slices of red onions and ginger (Note: take a dropperful of
  the wild greens drops (i.e. GreensFlush) to detoxify the
  mercury)
- Papaya Sprouts Salad With Avocado*
- Fried Eggplant with Yogurt*
- Bowl blueberries or blackberries in heavy cream or whole milk

Day 4

Breakfast
- Mediterranean Fried Eggs*

- Large glass fresh-squeezed grapefruit juice
- herbal tea with wild oregano honey

Lunch
- Sour Organic Chicken Stir Fry*
- Baked potato with real organic butter and organic sour cream
- Papaya 'n Kiwi Arugula Salad*

Dinner
- Organic Steak with Fried Leeks*
- Buttered Wild Shrimp*
- Pumpkinol-Dressed Chopped Salad*
- Melon or sliced kiwi fruit

Day 5

Breakfast
- Ground organic turkey patty or turkey sausage. Eat with mustard
- Bowl oat bran cereal topped with crude raw honey and real cream or whole milk
- Glass fresh-squeezed orange or tangerine juice
- Tablespoon cold-pressed walnut or hazelnut oil

Lunch
- Papaya 'n Kiwi Arugula Salad*
- Pomegranate Surprise*
- Large ground beef patty; top with cheese and eat with mustard and unsweetened ketchup (i.e. Westbrae's Unketchup)

Dinner
- Unbelievable Kenyan Lamb Stew*
- Mediterranean Tomato Salad*

- Herbal tea with raw oregano honey
- Honey Nut Wild Berry Dessert*

Day 6

Breakfast
- Nutri-Sense shake
- 1/2 grapefruit
- 1 boiled egg, as soft as possible
- WildPower Tea

Lunch
- Extra-Ordinary Beef 'n Vegetable Soup*
- Yogurt-Eggplant Puree´*
- Bowl strawberries or mixed berries; top with sugar-free whipped heavy cream (or add a bit of honey to sweeten, if desired)

Dinner
- Mediterranean Meat Loaf*
- Baked squash or sweet potato
- Mixed greens salad with plenty of sliced radishes and turnips
- Vintage (1940s) French Dressing*
- Glass of tomato or V-8 Juice

Day 7

Breakfast
- Bowl brown rice cereal; top with Nutri-Sense and whole milk; add crude raw honey for taste
- 2 poached eggs
- Glass fresh-squeezed grapefruit juice

Lunch
- Simple Sardine chopped Salad*
- glass tomato juice
- Purée of Turnip Soup*

Dinner
- Roast beef drizzled with Pomegranate Syrup
- Home-made mashed potatoes (or baked potato)
- Cucumbers With Dill and Sour Cream*
- Curried Vegetables*
- Blueberries with whipped cream and raw honey

Day 8

Breakfast
- Naturally-raised elk, turkey, or chicken sausages
- Bowl oat bran cereal (top with tablespoon nut oil)
- Pomegranate Surprise (2 tablespoons Pomegranate Syrup in spring or sparkling water on ice)

Lunch
- Huge mixed greens salad topped with organic full-fat cottage cheese and raw sunflower or pumpkin seeds; drizzle with extra virgin olive oil and vinegar.
- Mixed diced melon
- Glass mineral water

Dinner
- Mediterranean Meatballs With Pine Nuts*
- Brussels sprouts in butter or extra virgin olive oil
- Baked sweet potato (drizzle with crude pumpkinseed oil)
- freshly squeezed grapefruit juice
  (aids in the digestion of meat)

Day 9

Breakfast
- Egg 'n Onion Souffle*
- Glass V-8 juice; add one or two tablespoons Nutri-Sense
- Tablespoon Pumpkinol

Lunch
- Chopped variety root salad, containing parsnips, parsley root, green onions, turnips, and radishes (smothered with Pumpkinol)
- Old-Fashioned Muligatawny Soup*
- Lemon or lime water

Dinner
- Simple Curried Chicken*
- Steamed broccoli or cauliflower (both are high in naturally occurring vitamin C; if there is any juice remaining in the cooking fluids, drink it or use for soup)
- Wild rice or 50/50 wild and brown rice mixture; add in during cooking a few capsules of OregaMax and HerbSorb

Day 10

Breakfast
- Bowl full-fat organic cottage cheese (top with Nutri-Sense and diced melon of your choice)
- Glass grapefruit juice
- 1 to 2 boiled eggs
- Tablespoon cold-pressed hazelnut oil

Lunch
- Fresh wild fish of any kind; squeeze a full lemon over it (note: lemon helps detoxify heavy metals, such as mercury, which is a contaminant in most fish)
- Curried Vegetables*
- Tea with sliced ginger

Dinner
- Beef and Green Bean Stew*
- Steamed collards or kale topped with lemon and butter
- Wild rice
- Enzyme-Rich Fruit and Cottage Cheese Delight*
- Currant-C (organic mountain-grown currant juice)

Day 11

Breakfast
- Oat bran cereal topped with Nutri-Sense; add cream or whole milk plus raw honey, nuts, and seeds.
- Organic turkey, chicken, or venison sausages (nitrate-free)
- Glass fresh-squeezed orange juice
- Tablespoon Sesam-E

Lunch
- Nut butter sandwich on coarse whole grain bread; spread on butter and honey, if desired
- Beetroot and Olive Salad*

Dinner
- Grilled organic beefsteak, any type
- Grilled or raw onions
- Wild Rice and Nut Salad*

- Ghee-Fried Carrots*
- Pomegranate Surprise

Day 12

Breakfast
- Nut butters (but not peanut) on cheese and vegetables
- 1/2 cantaloupe or honeydew melon
- Wild Labrador Leaf Brew*

Lunch
- Simple Sardines in Salsa-Avocado Sauce*
- Steamed green beans or asparagus
- Glass V-8 juice

Dinner
- Hamburger (organic/grass fed-source) and vegetable casserole; top with cheese, if desired
- Baked squash topped with nut butter or real butter; add cinnamon (squash is high in potassium and pro-vitamin A, that is beta carotene)
- Famous Turkish Cucumber and Yogurt Salad*
- Sesame Seed Paste Surprise*

Day 13

Breakfast
- Nutri-Sense Super-Enriched Shake
  (mix 3 heaping tablespoons Nutri-Sense with whey protein and organic yogurt. Add a handful sunflower seeds or pine nuts. Add also raw honey and berries; blend, adding water to desired thickness)

- Ground buffalo or venison patty (sprinkle with OregaMax)
- Glass grapefruit juice or Pomegranate Surprise

Lunch
- Healthy Wild Tuna Salad*
- Oven-baked potatoes topped with parsley and spices; add organic sour cream or butter, if desired
- Lemon or lime water

Dinner
- Organic sirloin steak, medium or medium-rare
- Baked sweet potato topped with crude naturally pressed pumpkinseed oil (i.e. Pumpkinol) or nut butter
- Diced Enzyme-Rich Fruit Salad*
- Simple Sour Onion Salad*
- Currant-C in mineral water

Day 14

Breakfast
- Eggs Over Easy With Spices*
- Bowl oat bran cereal topped with Nutri-Sense, sliced almonds, and raw honey (i.e. wild oregano honey) and whole organic milk
- Glass fresh-squeezed grapefruit juice
- Tablespoon Oil of Wild Black Seed

Lunch
- Middle Eastern Spinach and Yogurt Soup*
- Salmon salad with diced vegetables, artichokes, cherry tomatoes, and olives (mix in crude pumpkinseed oil, i. e.

Pumpkinol, and balsamic vinegar) and contents of 2 or 3
OregaMax capsules
- Bowl Greek olives
- V-8 juice

Dinner
- Japanese Fresh Shrimp and Vegetables*
- Tossed dark green salad with spicy greens like watercress,
  mustard greens, and arugula; add feta cheese, if desired.
- Simple Middle Eastern Salad Dressing*
- Wedge melon or pineapple (note: the latter has antiseptic
  enzymes, but only when fresh)

Now you have it. These are special menus, which help
boost the immune system. Many of the foods on these menus
contain germ-killing components. This aids in the reversal of
high blood pressure as well as heart disease. The primary
germicidal foods or food components include the Pumpkinol,
raw honey, especially the Wild Oregano Honey, fatty fish oils,
lemon, lime, papaya and its seeds, fresh pineapple, hard kiwi,
onion, garlic, oregano, radishes, turnips, extra virgin olive oil,
and vinegar. All such substances help the the body kill germs.
Plus, these foods strengthen cellular health, greatly increasing
the resistance against disease.

Pay particular attention to the sesame seed paste recipes.
The fact is sesame seed extracts have been shown to help
normalize blood pressure. The regular inclusion of sesame
seed paste, fortified with the Sesam-E, will greatly aid
cardiovascular health. At every breakfast, ideally, some type
of nut or seed oil should be consumed, the emphasis being oils
of wild black seed and sesame.

There is plenty of protein in these menus, which is needed
for cellular strength and repair. The food is nutrient-dense,

which greatly increases overall resistance. Regarding meat sources only organic or grass-fed sources must be consumed. For fish only the wild types must be eaten. Farm-raised fish have up to 14 times more toxins than the truly wild types. By selecting healthy meats this will reduce the infection load placed upon the body. Regarding milk products and eggs it is crucial to consume only organic sources. Corrupt farming practices are the cause of disease, even epidemics. By purchasing only truly naturally raised animal products this encourages changes in the industry. This is how the private person can make a statement. Your shopping dollars do make a difference.

Healthy food helps keep the body in ideal condition, increasing the resistance to disease. When a plague strikes, resistance is the difference between disease and health, even life and death. The need for increased resistance is paramount. People are dying, and little is being done about it. Through the powers of nature and proper healthy diet innumerable lives could be saved.

Peoples' health is being systematically degraded. Toxins of all sorts have overwhelmed the human body, greatly diminishing its powers. Even today the food is largely poisonous. This is why people are suffering from a wide range of chronic diseases, largely due to weakened immunity. Yet, ultimately, such diseases are due to toxic exposure.

The immune system is highly susceptible to toxins. In fact, it is its very job to deal with them. The increased toxic load places such a great burden upon the immune system, that it is rendered dysfunctional. Yet, peoples' health could be dramatically improved strictly by making radical changes in the diet, by systematically cleansing such toxins and by taking the appropriate nutritional supplements.

Chapter 8

The Treatment Plan

For every disease it is crucial to have a strategic plan for its reversal. Here, in addition to diet nutritional supplements play a crucial role. This is certainly true of high blood pressure as well as heart disease. Most people follow a kind of haphazard approach, taking advice or ideas from a wide range of sources. What follows are systems that reverse the cause of hypertension, based upon years of experience. Only the most unprocessed natural substances are used, replete with the biological energy capable of curing. It is the North American Herb & Spice Company which produces such supplements.

Even so, each person is different in size, sensitivities, and overall body chemistry. However, some general rules apply to all. This is in regard to the antiseptic purge. For all hypertensive individuals it is crucial to purge the body of all infections, especially those entering the bloodstream. It is also crucial to solidify the health of the gums and teeth, which can also be achieved supplementally as well as through proper diet. A dental hygiene plan is also crucial.

The following are the supplements, which aggressively reverse this condition, in other words, which root out the cause. Rather than for mere nutritional replacement they are for eradicating this condition. This can be done by thoroughly supplying the cells with the nutrients they need. This can be accomplished through the regular intake of whole food concentrates.

SUPPLEMENT PLAN FOR HYPERTENSION

This is a specific plan to eradicate this condition. The purpose is to eliminate, that is reverse, the cause. In any such plan the key is patience. There may be temporary challenges in any new approach, minor hurdles to overcome. For instance, in some individuals as a result of taking supplements the blood pressure might temporarily rise. This is particularly true of oil of wild oregano, which increases the pumping power of the heart. However, this should fail to be a cause of alarm. Consistently following the supplement program is the answer, again, the key is consistency.

All spices improve the heart's pumping power. When this occurs, the heart must pump against stiffened, that is scarred and diseased, arteries. Thus, there may be a spike in the blood pressure. However, from an herbal medicine point of view this is no need for concern. The fact is as the oregano eradicates hidden infections, the health of the arteries will normalize and, thus, the blood pressure will correspond. Plus, it takes time to regenerate the arteries as well as the heart. The key is to destroy the infection, and wild oregano is the primary substance for achieving this. For aggressive action take both the oregano oil under the tongue and the OregaBiotic capsules orally.

Natural medicines cannot harm or destroy the body. Only drugs do that. Thus, regardless of any challenges stick with it. This is the only way you can ultimately rid yourself of this plague. The treatment plan is divided into three protocols, based upon severity:

Mild Hypertension

- OregaBiotic: two capsules twice daily with a full meal. For people with sensitive stomachs take capsules with a tablespoon or two of extra virgin olive oil with every dose
- Oreganol P73: three or more drops under the tongue twice daily
- Resvital crude red sour grape: three capsules twice daily or if taking the powder, a heaping teaspoonful twice daily
- Garlex true cold-pressed garlic complex: 10 drops twice daily in juice or water or under the tongue
- CranFlush (as a natural diuretic) 5 to 10 drops twice daily in juice or water or under the tongue

Moderate Hypertension

- OregaBiotic: two capsules twice daily with a full meal. For people with sensitive stomachs take capsules with a tablespoon or two of extra virgin olive oil
- Oreganol P73: ten drops under the tongue twice daily
- Resvital crude red sour grape: three capsules three times daily or if taking the powder, two heaping teaspoonfuls twice daily
- CranFlush wild berry drops (from wild high bush cranberries and wild purple berries): 40 drops twice daily under the tongue or in juice/water
- Garlex true cold-pressed garlic complex: 20 or more drops twice daily in juice or water or under the tongue.
- Hyper-Ten blood pressure-lowering herbal combination— three capsules twice daily
- Resvital powder: take a heaping teaspoon twice daily

Severe Hypertension

- OregaBiotic: three capsules three times daily with a full meal—for people with sensitive stomach take capsules with a tablespoon or two of extra virgin olive oil
- Oreganol P73: 20 drops under the tongue twice daily
- Resvital crude red sour grape: four capsules three times daily or if taking the powder, a heaping tablespoon twice daily
- CranFlush wild berry drops (from wild high bush cranberries and wild purple berries): 20 or more drops twice daily under the tongue
- Juice of Oregano: a half ounce twice daily. Improves the pumping power of the heart and, thus, helps improve blood flow to all tissues. This may cause a temporary rise in blood pressure, followed by a normalization
- Garlex true cold-pressed garlic complex: 40 or more drops twice daily in juice or water or under the tongue
- WildPower Tea: follow instructions on label; two cups twice daily
- Resvital powder: take one or more teaspoons twice daily
- Infla-eez enzyme purging formula: 3 capsules three times daily taking care to consume if possible on an empty stomach
- Hyper-Ten blood pressure-lowering herbal combination—three capsules twice daily
- CardioClenz: combination of essential oils specifically for decontaminating the arteries, 10 to 20 drops twice daily

Extremely Severe Hypertension

- OregaBiotic: three capsules three times daily with a full meal—or people with sensitive stomachs take capsules with a tablespoon or two of extra virgin olive oil
- Oreganol P73: 20 to 40 drops under the tongue twice daily
- Resvital crude red sour grape: six capsules three times

daily or if taking the powder, a heaping tablespoon three times daily (see note below)

- CranFlush wild berry drops (from wild high bush cranberries and wild purple berries): 60 or more drops three times daily under the tongue or in juice/water
- Juice of Oregano: a half ounce twice daily. Improves the pumping power of the heart and, thus, helps improve blood flow to all tissues. This may cause a temporary rise in blood pressure, followed by a normalization
- Garlex true cold-pressed garlic complex: 40 or more drops three times daily in juice or water or under the tongue
- WildPower Tea: follow instructions on label; three cups twice daily
- Resvital powder: take a heaping tablespoon three times daily
- Infla-eez enzyme purging and antiinflammatory formula (inflammation is a cause of heart disease): 3 to 5 capsules three times daily taking care to consume if possible on an empty stomach
- Hyper-Ten blood pressure-lowering herbal combination: 5 or more capsules twice daily
- CardioClenz: combination of essential oils specifically for decontaminating the arteries, 20 to 30 drops twice daily

Note: for all people who have diabetes or Syndrome X add to the supplement protocol Oregulin as follows: for mild hypertension take one capsule twice daily, for moderate, one capsule with each meal, for severe, two capsules with each meal, and for extreme, three capsules with each meal. Be aware that Oregulin is a natural insulin-like agent, so for those who are taking insulin proceed with caution and be sure to monitor blood glucose levels. This is because Oregulin effectively lowers blood sugar levels. What's more, if the cholesterol is high, take also Cholestamin, 2 capsules twice daily.

Since it is a spice and since spices elicit strong responses in sensitive people oregano products may initially create a rise in blood pressure. This is nothing to fear. It is only temporary, and it cannot cause any harm. To avoid this take the oregano with a full meal, particularly a meal heavy in fat. This will drive the oregano oil into the lymphatics, where it is most effective. Ideally, take it along with a shot glass of extra virgin olive oil. This largely eliminates any temporary blood pressure rise. Even so, in contrast to drugs there is no danger of a harmful reaction. In other words, spice oils can't cause a heart attack, stroke, or death. This is true only of the edible spice oils made by North American Herb & Spice, for instance. The fact is human trials have proven that the edible oil of wild oregano, Oreganol P73, is non-toxic and is even safe for individuals with liver or kidney damage, since it combats inflamation.

Also, for the three aforementioned categories optional supplements are fish oils, folic acid, vitamin B_{12}, pyridoxine, riboflavin, magnesium, potassium, chromium, selenium, and calcium. Many of these substances are found in the Nuke Protect, which is part of the arterial cleansing plan. Even so, compared to the power of spice extracts vitamins and minerals have a relatively minor impact. Thus, for reversing heart and arterial disease the wild foods and food extracts such as spice oils, wild raw kelp, wild raw greens, wild raw berries, enzymes, garlic oil, and similar crude unprocessed substances are the most effective.

PLAN FOR HYPERTENSIVE CRISIS

In this event the intake of supplements must be aggressive. Natural cures are equally effective for this as they are for chronic high blood pressure. The key is high doses and aggressive therapy.

- Infla-eez: one or two capsules every half hour or hour until improvement is noted taken on an empty stomach; for small-framed individuals two capsules three times daily.
- Resvital powder: a heaping teaspoon several times daily; if using the capsules take three capsules every few minutes, that is until improvement is noted
- BerriesFlush berry powerdrops: two or more full droppers under the tongue twice daily every few minutes or every half hour or hour
- GreensFlush wild greens powerdrops: several drops under the tongue every few minutes or every half hour or hour
- Oreganol oil of wild oregano: a few drops under the tongue two or three times daily
- Garlex true cold-pressed garlic complex: 60 or more drops three to five times daily in juice or water or under the tongue
- Wild Oregano Honey: in some cases this is highly effective; wild raw honey is calming and helps maintain blood volume. Only the Wild Oregano Honey has proven effective for this condition. Take a teaspoon several times daily.
- Hyper-Ten blood pressure-lowering herbal combination: 3 or more capsules several times daily

SUPPLEMENT PLAN FOR ARTERIOSCLEROSIS

PLAN FOR ARTERIAL CLEANSING (roto-rooter or dissolving action plus toxin-cleansing action)

- Infla-eez: three capsules three or more times daily on an empty stomach; for small framed individuals two capsules three times daily. For large framed individuals four capsules three times daily may be necessary
- Wild greens drops (i.e. GreensFlush): two full droppers under the tongue twice daily

- BerriesFlush wild berry drops: two or more full droppers under the tongue twice daily
- Oreganol oil of wild oregano: ten drops under the tongue twice daily
- OregaBiotic: two or three capsules twice daily with food or juice
- Resvital powder: a heaping teaspoon twice daily; for large framed individuals take two heaping teaspoons twice daily
- Juice of oregano: an ounce twice daily; this helps increase the pumping power of the heart
- NukeProtect: potent cleansing action of raw kelp and potassium iodide, as well as organic selenium, take three capsules twice daily; for tough cases increase the dose, that is four to five capsules twice daily
- Purely-C: three or more capsules twice daily
- Garlex true cold-pressed garlic complex: 60 or more drops three to five times daily in juice or water or under the tongue
- Hyper-Ten blood pressure-lowering herbal combination: 3 or more capsules several times daily
- CardioClenz: combination of essential oils specifically for decontaminating the arteries, 10 to 20 drops twice daily

Note: The aforementioned programs are ideal for anyone with heart or arterial disease. Cleansing in the circulatory system means largely the killing of germs, plus the destruction of any inflammation as well as inflammatory plaques. There are some 60,000 miles of blood vessels in the body, and for optimal health to occur all must be regenerated and maintained. This is why a wide range of supplements are recommended. Healing is achieved through the natural vitamin C supplements, as well as the crude red grape. The blood flow is improved through the crude red grape plus enzyme therapy. The wild greens drops (i.e. GreensFlush) cleanses toxins, particularly heavy metal. It does so by cleansing heavy metal residues from the liver and brain. The antioxidant powers of the crude red grape plus the spice oils help protect the arterial and heart walls, as well as their muscles, from oxidative damage. All phases are covered by this plan. This is essentially the same plan as that for high blood pressure. All supplements are available from finer health food stores and naturally oriented pharmacies, or call 1-800-243-5242.

THE DENTAL PLAN

The health of the teeth and gums is critical regarding all forms of heart disease. That dental disease has a direct impact upon the circulatory system is undeniable. Price, in his monumental monograph, *Dental Infections and the Degenerative Diseases*, has clearly proven the link, that is that dental infections directly lead to infections, as well as disease, of the heart and arteries. Thus, to reverse any circulatory disease the dental issue must be resolved.

The health of the bones, which hold the teeth, and this includes the upper and lower jaw bones, is also critical. If these bones are weak and disease becomes established, this will damage the circulatory system. This is because such an infection creates vast disruption in immune function, effectively repressing it. Such a bone infection, which is highly common in Americans, particularly those who have endured repeated invasive dental procedures, is a primary cause of ill health.

The toxins, as well as germs, from such a site may be continually seeded into the blood. This may lead to a wide variety of diseases, including heart disorders, mitral valve prolapse, enlarged heart, pericarditis, endocarditis, kidney disease as well as arthritis and fibromyalgia. Regarding infection in the heart or heart valves one warning sign is a kind of hemorrhage that occurs under the nail-bed. This appears as difficult-to-see tiny splinter, and this is why it is called a splinter hemorrhage. In the extreme it may arise as tiny hemorrhages on the tips of the fingers or thumb. Another warning is shortness of breath under minimal exertion such as climbing a flight or two of steps. In order for the disease to be cured, the site of infection must be cleansed.

This does not mean a person must make frequent trips to the dentist. In some instances that could be counterproductive. This is because if there is chronic infection of the arteries and/or heart, invasive dentistry will aggravate it. So, this plan describes a non-invasive treatment for the teeth and gums.

Gum disease, as well as disease or caries of the teeth, is the heart's curse. Every time a person with such disease chews or brushes the teeth a bolus of infection is sent into the bloodstream. Just imagine what happens with invasive gum surgery or a tooth extraction. Dental fillings and root canals are even worse. These procedures drive the germs upwards towards the brain. I have traced certain cases of brain disease, for instance, multiple sclerosis, Parkinson's disease, ALS, and Alzheimer's disease, to invasive dentistry.

The dentist's drill drives the sepsis directly upwards against gravity. The germs enter the blood and lymphatics and are carried directly to the brain, where they create untold havoc. Thus, it is important to destroy any oral sepsis, since the internal organs themselves are at risk. The heart, lungs, brain, liver, and kidneys all can be readily damaged by mouth-based germs—and outright disease can form, even cancer—that is unless the germ counts are kept under control and any pockets of infection are eradicated.

The health will improve dramatically as a result of oral cleansing. This involves the proper mechanical cleaning of the teeth, particularly non-invasive methods. It may surprise certain people but flossing, while invaluable, can disseminate germs, since it is a relatively traumatic technique. So can simple tooth brushing, especially vigorous brushing using stiff bristles. There is much proof that aggressive brushing with the typical synthetic bristle-based toothbrush damages the gum line, even causing receding. This causes germs to enter the blood, plus the recession allows pockets of germ growth in the mouth. Thus, aggressive brushing may do more harm than good.

There are two brushing devices which are acceptable: one is mechanical and the other is natural. The mechanical device that wins my approval is the Rotadent. This is the only 'synthetic' brush I use. It is a rotary brush, the brush head being made of relatively soft material: nylon. The rotary motion is far less traumatic than the typical up and down uncontrolled motion of standard tooth-brushing. Used properly the trauma to the gums is nil, while the cleaning action is far superior to standard brushing. I put a drop or two of the Oreganol P73 on the head of the brush. Note: be sure to clean the inside of this device periodically; it accumulates dental crud. The Rotadent is a professional device and can only be ordered by a registered dentist. For more information regarding a dentist near you who can order the device call contact:

Rotadent
P. O. Box 3749
Batesville, Arkansas
1-870-698-2300

There is another technique/device that is even less traumatic. This is a plant stem known as the miswak or peelu stick. Miswak is an Arabic word. Peelu is an Urdu word. Thus, obviously this stick is found largely in the Middle and Far East. It is the twig of a tree. The brush was popularized by the

Prophet Muhammad, who was an enormous fan of dental hygiene. He recommended the miswak and the toothpick as well as regular use of water to rinse food and poisons out of the mouth. The miswak is highly aromatic. The bark is relatively soft and scrapes off easily, leaving a soft bristle. The bristles contain natural substances, which cleanse and sterilize the teeth and gums, in fact, the entire mouth. When using the miswak, oral odors are reduced, as is plaque. There is a substance within it which, apparently, helps strengthen the gums, reversing swelling and bleeding. Plus, compared to commercial brushes the miswak is non-traumatic to the gum tissues. To order a package of miswaks call 1-800-243-5242. Currently, these are not available in stores.

Many people are interested in germ killers for use in the mouth. Germ-killing mouth washes and hydrogen peroxide are examples. Neither of these approaches are ideal. Hydrogen peroxide, while killing germs, oxidizes the gum tissues, eventually causing severe damage. With chemical antiseptics germ resistance is inevitable. This is not the case with natural antiseptics. Such antiseptics kill germs, while, in fact, strengthening the tissues.

The Oreganol is a potent germ killer. Hundreds of case studies demonstrate another phenomenal benefit: strengthening and tightening of gum tissues. Dentists are rather shocked by the appearance of Oreganol-treated mouths. The gum tissues are firmly against the teeth, and pockets of infection are eradicated. The gums are healthy, strong, firm, and pink. Similar results can be gained through the highly specialized formula, OregaDENT. As a mouth cleanser that you swish and swallow, the Juice of Oregano may be used. This is a duo approach to keeping the gums in ideal condition: without toxicity.

Flossing is also important, as is using toothpicks. I prefer a natural, that is wood, toothpick over flossing, due to the rather aggressive action of the floss against the gums. However, there is a safe way to floss. Simply place a drop of Oreganol on the (clean) finger. Rub the Oreganol over the floss, and then use the Oreganol treated floss. This will minimize the flossing-induced spread of germs and will largely prevent flossing-induced gum infections. Remember, flossing breaks gum tissue. Then, there is bleeding. The open blood vessels readily absorb germs and these germs may readily enter the systemic circulation. The Oreganol or OregaDENT treatment helps prevent this.

Juice of wild oregano is the ideal mouthwash It is completely natural without any synthetic chemicals, not even flavorings or sweeteners. Simply hold about a half ounce of the juice in the mouth for as long as possible; swish about or gargle; swallow if possible. The juice provides natural forms of oxygen in the form of oxygenated terpenes. These compounds are highly active against noxious oral germs, plus the oxygen helps nourish and strengthen the gums. The oxygenated terpenes have another unique property: penetration. They are solvent-like, so they are even capable of penetrating the enamel to root out deep-seated germs. For additional power a dropperful or two of OregaDENT may be added. Thus, the oral hygiene program is as follows:

- Oreganol oil (or OregaDENT) rubbed topically on the gums twice daily and/or added to the Rotadent
- The use of the soft-bristled natural toothbrush, that is the miswak
- Flossing, using floss, which is saturated with either the Oreganol or OregaDENT
- Toothpicks, especially after meals—note: you can soak the toothpick in the OregaDENT.
- The Juice of Oregano as a mouth cleanser

This protocol greatly strengthens the gums and teeth. Your dentist will know immediately. In fact, he or she will be shocked at the results and will ask you what you are doing. So will your doctor, because your overall health will dramatically improve.

INTERNAL CLEANSING PLAN

For vital health the body must be purged of all toxins. Such toxins irritate the nerves and, in fact, poison the nervous tissues, including the brain. If the toxins accumulate to a certain degree, high blood pressure results. Thus, in any high blood pressure treatment plan it is essential to remove the toxins. This plan is based upon the use of potent natural substances, which purge toxins from the deep tissues, that is from the cells and internal organs. The toxins are then flushed out of the body through the intestines and kidneys as well as through the pores of the skin.

Flush/Cleanse Plan
- GreensFlush wild greens drops from wild greens: 40 drops twice daily
- BerriesFlush wild berries drops: 40 drops twice daily
- Infla-eez: three capsules twice daily on an empty stomach; for extreme cases take four capsules two or three times daily
- CranFlush (to cleanse toxins from the kidneys and blood): one dropperful twice daily
- Oil of wild oregano (Oreganol): 10 drops twice daily
- Juice of wild oregano: 1/2 ounce twice daily
- Garlex: 40 drops twice daily
- healthy bacteria, natural lactobacillus-plus (Health-Bac): 1/2 teaspoon once or twice daily in warm water

Topical Cleanse

Toxins can be purged through the skin. This is accomplished by the use of spice oils, that is as lymphatic system stimulants.

- Oil of wild oregano (P73 Oreganol), using ideally the SuperStrength, rub the skin vigorously towards the heart once or twice daily
- Skin Clenz: as a multiple spice and herb cleanser rub on skin towards heart once or twice daily
- Oreganol cream (ideal for any inflamed skin lesions): rub on inflamed or irritated region as needed. Use on face to open capillaries and nourish the skin (may feel tingly for a short time—this means capillaries are opening)

Note: the topical scrubbing works best after a hot shower or bath which opens up the pores. This method of application helps dramatically speed the healing/cleansing response.

Chapter 9

Foods That Cure: The Recipes

On this plan food serves as a medicine. The recipes in this book are filled with ingredients rich in naturally occurring fats and spices. This is based upon the latest science. The fact is all the investigations to date have proven that in societies where large amounts of naturally occurring fats are consumed hypertension is unknown. In other words, in societies which avoid consuming synthetic fats, such as margarine, heart disease is essentially unknown.

Researchers often quote the example of the people in Finland as proof of the dangers of fats. In Finland heart disease, as well as hypertension, are epidemic. The Finns eat a significant amount of fat, including animal fat. However, what these investigators failed to reveal is that they also eat loads of synthetic fat: margarine, shortening, and hydrogenated oils, plus breads, pastries, cookies, cakes, chocolates, etc., which are contaminated with such oils. What's more, throughout

Scandinavia sugar consumption is at an all-time high. Furthermore, the Finns are notorious drinkers and smokers. Rather than natural fat consumption is these latter factors which play a far greater role in the onset of heart and arterial disease. In contrast, the Caucasus Russians, eat a more primitive diet and thrive on animal fat-rich foods without heart disease. The same is true of the Masai tribesmen, as well as the mountain-dwelling Turks. Neither the Turks or Caucasus Russians exercise regularly, other than walking. Thus, diet plays the primary role in prevention.

There are numerous other societies where high blood pressure and various forms of heart disease are rare: for instance, the Indian and the remote Pakistani tribes, the primitives of Sri Lanka, the natives of the Polynesian Islands, the mountain dwellers of Afghanistan. All have one thing in common: the regular use of spices. The fact is in any society where strong spices are regularly used heart disease is essentially unknown.

The ideal fats for this plan may surprise certain people. They are not the typical vegetable oils. Canola oil, which is genetically modified, is disqualified. Of course, extra virgin olive oil is a mainstay. Yet, so is butter, that is from organic sources. Palm kernel oil and virgin coconut oil are another invaluable category.

Virgin coconut oil has recently become popular. This is largely due to recent scientific studies which have demonstrated its beneficial properties. There is a special kind of coconut oil available, which is far superior to the commercial type. Known as cocapalm, this is a blend of the finest extra virgin coconut oil, plus wild spice oils. CocaPalm is a rich-tasting spread and may be used as a butter replacement. It is superior to butter for cardiovascular health.

The wild spice oils help give CocaPalm a rich robust flavor. Furthermore, these spices help protect the oil from oxidizing but, more importantly, protect the body from the oxidative effects of heated oil. CocaPalm is vastly superior to coconut oil alone. To order CocaPalm check finer heath food stores or call 1-800-243-5242. Thus, in summary the preferred oils are extra virgin olive oil, pure organic butter, and spice-enhanced coconut/palm oil. These are the richest tasting oils available. Yet, they are heart- and artery-safe. Other excellent oils for cooking include cold-pressed sesame oil, which is unfiltered (i.e. Sesam-E), hazelnut oil, grapeseed oil, and avocado oil.

Then, there are the salad oils, that is oils, which cannot be heated. These include cold-pressed flaxseed oil and pumpkinseed oil. Such oils readily oxidize, so they are unfit for heating or cooking. They may be added to soups at the end of cooking. The crude pumpkinseed oil is particularly valuable, due to its rich content of nutrients. It is a top source of naturally occurring vitamin E, plus it is high in chlorophyll. Incredibly, a mere tablespoon contains 10 I.U. of crude, unprocessed vitamin E. When fortified with antioxidant essential oils, it has a reasonably long shelf life. Such fortified pumpkinseed oil, known as Pumpkinol, is the ideal salad oil. As a salad oil a 50/50 mix of Pumpkinol with extra virgin olive oil or sesame seed oil is also acceptable.

On this plan, Mediterranean, as well as southeast Asian, recipes are emphasized. There is a specific reason for this. In these regions the incidence of heart and circulatory diseases is much lower than, for instance, in North America or Europe. This is largely because of the extensive use of novel foods and spices. The spices may play the most predominant role. Modern research is finding that of all foods spices have the most powerful of all biochemical profiles. In other words, the chemicals in spices offer the greatest protective powers of any natural substances. Here is the point: wherever spices are extensively consumed the incidence of heart and circulatory disease plummets. The following section is a brief introduction to the major spices and their uses.

Spices: medicines in your kitchen

It is time to rediscover the spice shelf, that is to understand the main spices and their uses. Recent research points to the medicinal powers of spices as being more powerful than any other group of plants, including herbs. In particular, spices have been shown to be powerful germ killers, as well as antioxidants. These antioxidant powers are particularly impressive.

An antioxidant is a substance which blocks oxidation. When exposed to the elements, a nail rusts, that is when exposed to oxygen. The same occurs within the human body. Antioxidants block such reactions, acting as cellular preservatives. ORAC testing proves that of all herbs and natural substance spices have the highest antioxidant powers. Vitamin E and beta carotene are relatively weak compared to the antioxidant strength of spices.

The oils of these spices are far more powerful than the herbs. Clove proved most potent, followed by oregano, cumin, and cinnamon. Wild Oregano and cumin are more powerful than the commercial types. For human use as a medicine only the wild type must be consumed.

Today, people regard spices only as seasonings. Perhaps it is possible to change that thinking. Open a jar of cinnamon and breathe the aroma: sense the tingle. Experience the dominating taste. That is its medicinal powers. The fact is cinnamon is a medicine, not merely a spice. Recent research documents its effects. It has been determined that the daily intake of a quarter teaspoon of cinnamon daily greatly aids diabetics, that is by helping regulate blood sugar. Incredibly, it acts like a natural insulin. Thus, it is time to rethink the value of spices: as medicines with culinary benefits. Recently, an anti-diabetic product, a specialized extract of cinnamon, fenugreek, wild oregano, and wild cumin, has become available. Known as Oregulin, this spice oil concentrate is a powerful regulator of blood sugar levels. Tests at Georgetown University prove that Oregulin reduces blood sugar levels by 40%, while increasing insulin sensitivity. In other words, Oregulin helps make insulin work better. The insulin is more active—the body needs less to achieve its purpose. Oregulin is the most powerful natural insulin- and blood sugar-regulating formula known.

In the Middle Ages traders searched the whole then-known-world for spices. During this era spices were valued to a greater degree than gold or silver. The fact is spices were the most sought after, as well as fought after, cargo. Today, they are taken for granted. The fact is they are invaluable for superb health. This is true of the truly unprocessed natural types. Now, most spices are irradiated, which destroys much of their medicinal value. So, always opt for spices or spice-based medicines which are uncorrupted and non-irradiated.

Spices can be used in any food, even salads and desserts. Do not be shy in using them. Traditionally, they have been relied upon for flavoring soups, meat dishes, stews, and sauces. Cooking greatly enhances their powers, that is their flavor. Uncooked foods, such as salad dressings, fruit dishes, and juices, need time for the flavors to 'marry': any herbs and spices added to such dishes must be included several days before serving. There is no rule on their use, so experiment. According to Spice Islands' *Guide to Your Spice Shelf* the correct herb/spice formula for any food is an individual choice: what tastes right. "The seasoning," say the editors, "is not a science but, rather, an...art." Let the spicing of food be an art to your liking. That will deliver the greatest benefits.

Spices are derived from the bark, root, fruit, flower, or berry of certain plants, mostly tropical and sub-tropical. In the tropics the hot sun creates special kinds of foliage, which produce aromatic compounds. These aromatic compounds are concentrated in the aforementioned parts of the plants. In contrast, herbs are exclusively leaves, which are also usually aromatic. Certain seeds of these herbs are aromatic and, therefore, spice-like, for instance, the seeds of anise, caraway, fennel, and coriander. What's more, certain vegetables are spice-like, that is they are hot and aromatic. These true vegetables include leeks, garlic, onion, peppers, paprika, radish, and horseradish. All contain a certain amount of aromatic compounds, which are spicy or hot in taste. The following is a partial list of key spices found in nature:

Allspice

This is the only spice which originates in the Western hemisphere. A native of Jamaica, allspice was so-named because its aroma and taste are a sort of combination of cinnamon, cloves, and nutmeg. The best tasting allspice comes from Jamaica, while the type produced in Mexico and Central America is inferior. Allspice is a potent germicide and is capable of killing viruses, yeasts, mold, and bacteria. It is used particularly in sweet dishes, baking, and roasting. It is ideal for bread and rice stuffings. In America its greatest use is in baking. It is also used extensively for pickling.

Anise seed

A native of Asia Minor this herb has grown wild for untold centuries. It is still found in vast tracts in the wilderness, even high in the mountains. Anise is a licorice-like spice. As a medicine it strengthens the adrenal glands, and, thus, it increases strength and vitality. It also helps balance hormones. Here, it is useful for combating hot flashes as well as PMS.

As a flavoring it is useful in fruit dishes and salads. Mostly, it is used in sweets, breads, and rolls. Anise is an ideal herb for strengthening the adrenal glands. It also contains an anti-diabetic principle. The highest quality anise comes from Turkey.

Basil

A native of tropical Africa and Asia, basil has been used as a medicine for tens of thousands of years. It is well known as a digestive aid. There is significant folk use in combating headaches. It is mostly used in soups, salads, vegetable dishes, stir fry, and in egg dishes, especially omelets and quiche. Basil greatly aids in the digestion of high protein foods, particularly eggs and meat. It makes an interesting addition to roast beef or lamb.

Bay leaf

Bay leaves come from a tree, which grows in virtually any temperate climate. However, the truly aromatic type is a native of the Mediterranean. In fact, it is the leaf of an enormous bush, which may grow up to 40 feet tall. Bay was used extensively by the ancient Greeks and Romans, certainly in food, but, perhaps for many unknown uses, including beautification. It is best used in soups, poached fish, roasts, stews, wild game, and marinades. It may also be added to custard and creams, where it imparts into the fat an aromatic essence. Here, an edible oil of bay leaf is ideal. This oil of bay leaf may also be added to rich soups as well as spaghetti sauce.

Cinnamon

This is perhaps the most widely used and famous of all spices. It was so treasured in ancient times that it was equated as currency. There are a wide range of cinnamon barks, and the flavor varies greatly, depending upon the species and location. These types are Ceylon Cinnamon, Saigon Cinnamon (in fact, cassia), and Batavia Cassia. These plants differ botanically.

Cinnamon is harvested from the tree's shoots by stripping them of their bark. These strips are then dried. The strips may be sold as is, that is cinnamon sticks, or ground into the common spice. Cinnamon is used in a wide range of dishes and foods, including teas and cold drinks, puddings, custard, hot fruit recipes, rolls, buns, meat dishes, milk-based desserts, pickles, and relishes. In America it is the mainstay of the hot cereal breakfast. An oil of edible cinnamon is available. Made from the highest quality cinnamon/cassia bark this may be used as an alternative for flavoring as well as a germicide. However, this oil is powerful; only small amounts should be consumed, for instance, five drops at a time. To order edible oil of cinnamon call 1-800-243-5242.

Cloves

This is nature's most powerful antioxidant spice. In ancient and medieval times it was also the most valued one. Cloves are a flower, in fact, the unopened bud of a tall tropical tree. This is one of the most expensive of all tropical spices. Cloves have been used, traditionally, mainly in bakery. They make a great addition to hot cider, fruit drinks, and, certainly, brown and wild rice dishes. They may also be used to impart a rich flavor to roasts.

The medicinal properties of cloves derive largely from its antioxidant powers. However, cloves are also a powerful germ killer. Hulda Clark, in her book, *Cure for All Cancers*, relies upon them as a kind of purge, that is to kill potentially cancer-causing parasites. In East Indian folk medicine this is confirmed: the regular intake of cloves can cause the expulsion and/or death of worms, amebas, and other parasitic invaders. An oil of edible clove buds is available, which can be taken as an intestinal purge. It is also invaluable as a dental aid, that is to combat pain, tingling, and infection. This is different than the commercially available clove oil, which may be derived from the leaves. The oil from the leaves is inedible, while that derived from the flowering buds is completely safe. To order this oil call 1-800-243-5242.

Coriander

A famous spice in India this is little known in the United States. However, it is a major component of the more well known curry powder. A native of Asia Minor, it has grown wild in this region for tens of thousands of years. In fact, it has disseminated from this region, and now grows wild throughout much of Europe. This is a kind of biblical spice, with records showing usage by both Moses and Jesus. The Prophet Muhammad recommended it highly as a medicine for virtually any illness, particularly disorders of the digestive tract. Modern research proves it is a carminative, which means it prevents abdominal spasticity, gas, and discomfort.

Unfortunately, few Americans use this spice, other than in curried dishes. Yet, ground coriander could be easily used on any meat, poultry, or fish dish. By making use of this highly aromatic herb digestive disorders will noticeably improve. Coriander is an active ingredient of HerbSorb, a digestive aid formula based upon unprocessed spice extracts. This is the ideal herb and spice formula for normalizing digestion. HerbSorb has been found useful for hiatus hernia, heartburn, esophageal reflux, bloating, diarrhea, and excessive gas. For digestive support enzymes may also be necessary. The Oregacyn Digestive combines potent plant-source enzymes plus natural spice extracts. This combination is ideal for stubborn digestive disorders.

Cumin seed

In North America except in Mexican food, for instance, chili, cumin seed is rarely used. This is a tremendous deficit, that is for human health. This is because cumin seed is one of the most powerful natural medicines known.

Research documents its impressive powers. One study determined that cumin raised the levels in tissue of a highly protective enzyme, glutathione-S-transferase, some 700%. This means that cumin and, particularly, extracts of this seed are a major disease preventive. Glutathione-S-transferase is the key enzyme for the removal of toxic substances from the body. This may explain cumin's potent action on the liver: it is instrumental in helping reverse chemically induced or infection-induced liver damage. This is why it is an active ingredient of Oregacyn Liver, which has been recently shown to reverse liver damage in hepatitis C patients.

Cumin is highly pungent. Most people find it intolerable. Thus, supplements are the ideal way to consume it. Wild extract of cumin is available as Cuminol. It is also an active ingredient in Oregacyn capsules. The latter is used primarily for respiratory disorders. Other foods which blend well with the taste of cumin include hard cheeses, creamed cheese, cheese dips, eggs (i.e. Mexican-style omelets), and roasts.

Curry powder

Contrary to popular belief this isn't mainly made from the curry plant. Rather, it is a blend of six or more spices, including cumin, coriander, fenugreek, turmeric, ginger, pepper, dill, mace, cardamom, and cloves. This combination gives curry powder its rich and exotic flavor. There are numerous curry blends; each region of India has its own recipe. The fact is in

India there is a unique "curry blend" for virtually every dish. It is only here in the West that a single blend is used for all. Curry powder is an excellent digestive aid. It should be used to flavor as many dishes as possible. It is mainly used for stir fry, sauce-based dishes, creamed dishes, in deviled eggs, and in marinades for any baked meat, poultry, or fish. It may also be used to flavor home-made roasted nuts.

Dill weed

This rich source of trace minerals should be made use of in the home. Dill is particularly high in potassium, magnesium, and calcium. Chopped dill is an ideal addition to finalize flavor in soups and sauces. It may also be added to any soft cheese dip. Traditionally, it is used to flavor buttery fish dishes. It is an excellent addition to cole slaw and cucumber salads. When serving avocado always add chopped dill weed.

Dill weed, largely because of its rich content of minerals, is of great value for kidney function: it is one of the richest sources of potassium known. It is a mild diuretic, which is completely safe to use despite medication.

Fennel

It is believed that this plant originated from southern Europe, however, others place its origin in the mountains of Asia Minor. During the Middle Ages fennel was used mainly as a medicine. It was believed to be an important cure for eye disorders as well as female complaints. It was also highly esteemed for its strength-producing qualities. Today, fennel is used almost exclusively as a seasoning or food. Its medical properties have been seemingly long forgotten. It is used in meat ball, sausage, and meat roll dishes, even meat loaf. It makes an excellent addition to buttery potato dishes. It may be used to season fish broths or soups. An edible oil of fennel seed is available. This finds great use in the most important folk application for this seed: colic, digestive disorders, irritable colon, spasms, and gas. Edible oil of fennel is an outright cure for such conditions. What's more, it is a highly effective cure for intestinal worms, especially hookworms. Fennel is an active ingredient in the anti-parasitic product, Intesti-Clenz. This is a specific formula for stomach and intestinal disorders, for instance, nausea, vomiting, spastic stomach, stomachache, irritable bowel, and gas. The fact is such disorders are likely caused by intestinal, as well as liver, parasites, and Intesti-Clenz kills these. Intesti-Clenz is a potent formula for killing a wide range of parasites, including worms and protozoans. Made with wild fennel and cumin seed oils this is safe even for pets and children. It is also an active ingredient of the children's product, Kid-e-Kare Tumi-eez. The latter is ideal for any stomach or upper intestinal disorder in children. It is also more palatable than the Intesti-Clenz. To order the Intesti-Clenz or Kid-e-Kare Tumi-eez call 1-800-243-5242.

Garlic

Garlic saves lives. It can help keep people alive when all else fails. During the 1918 flu pandemic garlic was successfully used to ward off potentially fatal infections. This is one of the most powerful food-medicines known. Even so, there is a certain vulgarity about it. The smell of garlic on a person's breath is offensive. Raw garlic is somewhat harsh on the gut. Even so, regular garlic eaters benefit from its wide range of medicinal actions. Garlic kills the majority of noxious germs, including hidden parasites. It thins the blood and blocks arterial damage. It moderately lowers cholesterol levels.

Garlic, as well as garlic powder and salt, greatly add to the flavor of food. This is largely due to the highly flavorful sulfur compounds. The uses of this invaluable herb are legion, beyond the mention of this book. It makes a tasty addition to any cheese sauce or dip. In gravies it livens all tastes. Mixed in hamburger it protects against germs, while boosting digestion. Garlic helps speed the digestion of meat fat. Roasted along with steak it takes the heaviness away from the meat. However, again, beware: raw garlic can prove offensive. Never eat it when you must be close to others. If you do so, eat afterwards a few sprigs of parsley to minimize the odor. As a garlic oil supplement fortified with wild oregano oil consider Garlex. This is a means to gain the benefits of a cold-pressed garlic oil, which has never before been made available. The garlic is grown on rich soils in the Mediterranean, then the cloves are pressed by a time-tested ancient method. No heat is used in the process. Known as Garlex this is a mild tasting garlic-oregano oil, which can be added to food or juice. Or, it may be taken sublingually. Ideally, take it with fatty foods. To order call 1-800-243-5242.

Ginger

This is one of the most versatile of all spices. It adapts to virtually any food. In the United States it is perhaps most popular in sweets, bakery, and fish, although in the early part of this century ginger-based drinks were infamous.

Ginger is more of a medicine than a food. It contains a variety of potent chemicals, with a vast array of medicinal actions. These chemicals include a variety of substances which block inflammation. Ginger is also rich in natural antibiotics. Its use for digestive disorders is legendary, therefore the origin of Gingerale. Unfortunately, true ginger-based ales which are effective for reversing stomach disorders are unavailable. However, the edible oil is available. This is a cold-extracted ginger oil, a process which retains, in fact, potentiates, its medicinal actions. The edible oil is available as Oil of Ginger made by North American Herb & Spice Co. The fact is Oil of Ginger is a potent agent for reversing digestive disorders. Use it along with sparkling water and raw honey to make your own gingerale. To order cold-pressed ginger oil call 1-800-243-5242.

Horseradish

There could be no better health food than horseradish. Rather than a food this is a powerful medicine. All its power is derived from the chemicals responsible for its hot taste, which are due to specialized sulfur compounds as well as enzymes. Horseradish is rich in a special enzyme known as peroxidase. This is one of the most potent anti-cancer substances known. Peroxidase helps halt toxic reactions, known as free radical reactions, which damage the heart and arteries.

The importance of halting free radical reactions is often discussed. Yet, what is even more critical is determining the cause of such reactions. If the factors which are generating such reactions are corrected, this is more critical than merely quenching free radical reactions. What's more, it is infection which is largely responsible for such reactions. This is another benefit of the anti-infection protocol. It attacks the true cause. Thus, if the toxins and/or inflammation are eliminated, that is if the underlying infection is eradicated, then the free radical reactions are halted and the tissues can heal. Because of its potent content of infection- and inflammation-fighting enzymes horseradish can play a role in reversing circulatory diseases. Horseradish extract, in fact, the extract of the wild plant, is one of the active ingredients of Infla-eez. This helps halt oxidative reactions within the arteries, and it also helps the body destroy noxious invaders. Remember, an individual is only as healthy as his or her arteries. Infla-eez, rich in horseradish peroxidase, helps prevent arterial degeneration.

During the Middle Ages horseradish was a universal antidote. In Europe it was relied upon for virtually any illness. It was only during the late 1400s that it became popular with food.

Much of the medicinal properties of this plant are attributable to its family of origin: the mustard genus. Such plants are rich in a wide range of sulfur compounds which are directly toxic to cancer cells. Horseradish is also mildly antibacterial and antifungal. The fresh root is a good source of vitamin C and was used in 15th through 17th century Europe to cure scurvy. Currently, it is mainly used in fish sauces, a most appropriate venue, since it is germicidal and since it boosts protein digestion. It is also the ideal condiment for steaks, where, again, it is of great "digestive" value. When made into a cream sauce, it may be used as a dip for any grilled or roasted meat.

Mint

This is perhaps the most popular of all American spices, being used in so-called All-American fare such as lemonade, 'mints', chewing gum, and mint jelly (for leg of lamb). In ancient times it was highly regarded as a flavoring. The first mint sauce was made apparently in the 3rd century A.D. Incredibly, in ancient times it was used in tooth cleansing formulations. Today, the value of mint as a medicine is minimal, although some studies document a beneficial action on the colon, particularly for irritable bowel sufferers. What's more, mint allergy is relatively common. This can be manifested by stiff neck, headache, agitation, joint pain, stomachache, spastic colon, and hives. Even so, mint is a highly relaxing herb, especially when taken as a tea, that is made from the fresh leaves, along with raw honey. It is soothing as an after dinner tea, as it aids digestion. This herb is ideal for fresh fruit compotes, fruit juice, and all lamb dishes. Crushed, it may blend well with full fat cottage cheese.

Mustard

This is a highly stimulating spice, which has a diversity of uses. In the 1600s the famous Nicholas Culpeper observed that people who have difficulty digesting meat are cured through a mustard-cinnamon mixture. This is precisely the use for mustard today. Instinctively, people crave it on meats, particularly beef. What's more, mustard contains germ-killing chemicals. This may explain the early American use of mustard poultices for lung or chest infections.

Onions

Onions are perhaps the most ancient of all foods. They are also one of humankind's most ancient medicines. For instance, in ancient Rome onions were a staple, both as food and medicine. Roman warriors claimed that the ingestion of onions gave them greater strength in battle. Alexander the Great gave his soldiers a daily ration of it. Pliny the Elder documented the Roman use of this potent herb: to minimize wound infections, reverse diarrhea, eliminate toothache, and, when used as a suppository, for reversing hemorrhoids. Yet, this is no wives' tale. Dr. Leonard Pike, Texas A & M scientist, has documented the onion's medicinal powers. Chemicals in onions, claims Dr. Pike, halt free radical production, a major factor in the cause of degenerative disease. Onions contain a variety of chemicals with potent anti-cancer effects and, apparently, certain of these chemicals are particularly active in blocking the toxicity of carcinogens in the intestines. Extracts of onion stimulate enzymes, which detoxify carcinogens. The results indicate that the regular intake of this food may stall the development of digestive cancers, particularly colon cancer. According to Pike, "All that folk medicine...about the power of onions, has a basis in fact."

Onions are also beneficial for the circulatory system. Chemists at East Texas State University discovered a substance in onions, which lowers the blood pressure as well as thins the blood. Obviously, this would prove invaluable for high blood pressure victims. This blood thinning substance was extracted and used successfully in test animals. Investigators at George Washington University School of Medicine have found that onions contain a substance that blocks the formation of thromboxane, a chemical which causes blood to clot. Thus, this versatile food offers dependable blood-thinning actions. What's more, the regular intake of onions helps prevent excessive levels of blood fats. Experiments in India have demonstrated that onions help reduce dangerously high cholesterol levels.

The onion is the most versatile of all spices/herbs. It can be used in virtually every dish. It blends well in all soups, sauces, meat dishes, fish dishes, stews, eggs, cheeses, dips, and more. Due to its blood-thinning, as well as antiseptic, actions it is regularly included in this diet. What's more, it is an active ingredient of OregaMax capsules, the contents of which are added to many recipes.

Oregano

Unknown in this country until the 1950s oregano has become highly popular. However, its use is generally limited to Italian-style food, particularly pizza and spaghetti. This may largely be due to its source: much of the commercial oregano is from Mexico, where a kind of sage brush with an oregano-like taste is harvested. This is far more pungent than the truly Mediterranean oregano, which limits its use. Thus, the truly wild Mediterranean oregano is more versatile. It has a more subtle flavor than the Mexican type. This is the type used in this book. Common uses of oregano include the addition into salad dressings, tomato salads, spaghetti, meat sauces, roasts, zucchini, hot tomato dishes, eggplant dishes, and meat loaf.

One way to ensure that it is wild oregano is to buy the actual plant, that is the dried plant, stems and all. The villagers cut the oregano at the lower stems, and then dry the plant. The plant, being a perennial, regrows. These are known as oregano bunches. Of course, the wild oregano may also be found as a supplement, that is the OregaMax unprocessed wild herb capsules and the oil of wild Oreganol (P73). Regarding the latter these may be added to foods, particularly sauces, stir fry, roasts, and soups. The contents of one or more OregaMax capsules make a superb addition to cheese dips. Rubbed on roast or poultry carcass the oil helps tenderize the meat as well as season it. As a result of the Oreganol rub the meat tends to fall off the bone and is far less tough. Also, the seed from the wild-growing Mediterranean plant may be purchased: call 1-800-243-5242.

Paprika

The most mild of all spices paprika got its fame in Hungarian dishes: goulash is loaded with it. Early in the 1900s Americans developed a taste for paprika, although it has little taste. In fact, it is the color that is so attractive in garnishing food. Paprika is a top source of beta carotene. It may be added to virtually any dish. It should be added in higher quantities than it is currently used.

Parsley

This is one of the most invaluable vegetable/herbs known. It has one of the most ancient uses of any known food. In ancient Greece and Rome it was highly popular, both as food and garnish. The current use as a garnish derives from them. This is an insufficient use, that is as a mere garnish. The fact is its nutrient content is so rich that it should be eaten as a main course. Parsley is exceptionally high in magnesium, potassium, iron, vitamin C, and folic acid. Its rich supply of magnesium accounts for one of its prime benefits: its significant diuretic action. There are two components: the leaves and the root. The root is particularly pungent, and, while rarely used, makes an excellent raw vegetable for salads. It is also ideal as an addition to vegetable soups. The root tastes luscious when added to stews and roasts. It imparts a rich flavor to meat.

Pepper

I am not a major fan of pepper. It contains potentially toxic alkaloids. Commercial pepper is highly oxidized; only freshly ground pepper should be used. Occasionally, I have freshly ground black pepper over salads and meats. Of course, it is invaluable as a flavoring for mashed or roasted potatoes but, again, only the freshly ground type should be used. What's more, allergic intolerance to black pepper is common, which may result in skin rashes, swellings, sore throat, chest congestion, and headaches. It is readily evident that there is an enormous difference between freshly ground black pepper and the regular type. Regarding the latter it is often extended with additives for cost purposes. Thus, for health purposes only the freshly ground type must be used.

Red (hot) pepper

Black and red pepper are, botanically, unrelated. In contrast to black pepper the red or chili peppers have no aromatic oil. Rather, they depend upon rather caustic or irritating chemicals for their heat. This is why I don't make major use of it in my kitchen, preferring instead the more gentle, that is intestinally, herbs and spices such as oregano, cumin, sage, rosemary, paprika, parsley, onion, etc.

The problem is in many dishes hot pepper conceals other flavors. It overpowers many aromas. So, I rarely purposely add it to food, using it only when absolutely necessary. I simply don't like its overpowering effects, even though from a health point of view there is value. This overpowering effect can be minimized, that is by using only a tiny amount, essentially, as a flavor enhancer. In this instance the activating powers of hot pepper, in fact, enhance other flavors. This is particularly true in fat-rich dishes. What's more, the fat helps modify the peppery flavor and, thus, in fatty foods a greater amount can be added. Thus, the key with this herb is to avoid overusing it. As a digestive stimulant it can prove valuable. What's more, it has a mild action against heart disease by causing relaxation of the arteries. The major value of hot pepper is in heart disease. Here, as a vasodilator it is invaluable.

Rosemary

A highly pungent herb, rosemary was known in ancient times, for its medicinal properties. It was regarded as the herb-of-choice for mental disorders, including depression, anxiety, and, particularly, memory loss.

Rosemary is a powerful herb. Thus, it may overpower all other flavors. Americans use little of it; it is invaluable for health, and, thus, it should be used more extensively. It creates an addictive taste with chicken, especially if roasted with the skin on. The same is true of roast turkey and even roast beef. Of course, it is traditional to use rosemary with roast lamb. The regular use of rosemary with fatty meats helps improve fat digestion, while helping the body in the processing of animal fat. Rosemary blends well with fat and helps prevent fat-induced toxicity. It helps neutralize any toxicity that might be transmitted by the fats. Thus, it tastes good, while serving an invaluable biological function.

In American fare the uses are limited but growing. Now it is common to find old world-style breads with rosemary, especially olive bread. It is also added to quiche, omelets, and cheese dips. It is dusted or crumbled on scrambled or over-easy eggs.

Sage

There is an ancient proverb which claims that if a person regularly uses sage, no disease will afflict him. This is a sensible claim. The fact is recent research documents that sage is one of the most powerful cellular preservatives known. What's more, it contains antiviral properties, which match, in fact, exceed any drug. Sage has been long used to calm the nerves. Apparently, it contains a substance which enhances the natural production of specialized chemicals within the nerves known as neurotransmitters. Its main use is in stuffings, vegetable dishes, roasts, organ meats, poultry, and creamed soups. Sage blends particularly well in any dish which is fatty.

In these recipes there is also an emphasis on wild foods, that is as many wild foods as are readily available. In the common markets there are relatively few foods, which are truly wild, for instance, pine nuts, wild blueberries, wild rice, sardines, and similar options. Yet, for each person's benefit as many of these are incorporated into the recipes as possible. These are foods from the Highest Source available: the almighty Maker of this universe. Research has proven that wild foods are up to five times more potent in terms of nutritional value, as well as a source of antioxidants, than commercial sources. This proves the power of unaltered, that is the substances from almighty God, versus human corruptions.

So, spices should be consumed profusely. So should natural fats. What's more, as many wild foods as is possible should be eaten. As a result, your heart and arteries will become healthier, smoother, less scarred, less inflamed, and less diseased. The infections will dissipate, and you will be able to live a fuller and more vital life. That is a promise, a fact which nature, as well as civilization, has proven. So, eat with relish and gusto: enjoy. Your life will improve dramatically.

SIMPLE, POWERFUL RECIPES

No one has time to cook. Thus, the following are simple, that is fast, recipes that you can easily create in your kitchen. Many of these food items have been listed in the Two Weeks of Eating Right section.

Many of the forthcoming recipes contain fat, that is natural fat from healthy sources. Some of these fats are of animal origin: butter, whole milk, cheese, fish fat, poultry fat, and beef fat. There is no need for concern regarding such fats. Remember, the fat-eating primitives, the Inuit, Masai, Greeks, Turks, Caucasus Russians, Yemeni Jews, and countless others, rarely develop high blood pressure despite consuming fat-rich diets. They only develop this disease when following the Western diet. So, enjoy these recipes without concern. These foods will help lower or normalize blood pressure, never raise it.

Meat, Fowl, and Fish

High Blood Pressure-Beating Hamburger

1 lb. organic hamburger meat
1 medium to large yellow or red onion, diced
2-3 cloves organic garlic, diced
contents four to six OregaMax capsules
extra virgin olive oil

In a mixing bowl combine hamburger with onions, garlic, and contents of OregaMax capsules. In a skillet heat a small amount of olive oil over medium-low heat; add meat, molded into four-ounce patties. Cook to desired doneness, being careful not to overcook, since this destroys much of the nutritional value.

Mediterranean Meat Loaf

2 lb. minced organic lamb or beef
2 onions, finely minced (or, preferably, grated)
sea salt and freshly ground pepper
1 can organic tomato paste
butter as needed
4 tablespoons fresh parsley, minced
contents 4 OregaMax capsules
1 teaspoon freshly ground cinnamon sticks
1/4 teaspoon freshly ground allspice

Repeatedly mince meat. Add the grated onions and blend with meat until it all becomes a smooth paste. Season to taste with salt, pepper; add cinnamon, allspice, and contents of OregaMax capsules. Spread evenly over the bottom of large oiled or buttered baking tray, flattening out with a wooden spoon or spatula. The meat must be about an inch thick. In a preheated oven (375 degrees) bake until surface is browned: about 40 minutes. Mix tomato paste with 1/2 pint water and pour over meat. Return to oven and continue for 10 minutes or until sauce is well absorbed. Serve as squares or rounds. Garnish with fresh parsley and serve piping hot.

Mediterranean Meatballs with Pine nuts

2 lb. lamb or beef
1 teaspoon ground cinnamon or allspice

sea salt and freshly ground black pepper to taste
2 large yellow onions, cut in slices, then halved
organic butter as needed
2 1/2 oz. pine nuts
1 medium-sized can organic tomato concentrate (about 5 oz.)
teaspoon Resvital powder (or juice of half lemon)
3 tablespoons parsley, finely minced

Mince, pound, or knead meat to a smooth paste. Add seasoning. Knead well and roll into balls.

In a saucepan, fry onions gently in butter until golden. Add meatballs and sauté over low heat, shaking pan and rolling balls nearly constantly to color evenly. Add pine nuts and brown for 2 minutes (low heat). Mix tomato with a bit of water and add. Add more water, that is to cover balls; flavor with lemon or Resvital and season with more salt and pepper. Stir well and simmer until well done and sauce is reduced, but add water if sauce is over-reduced. Just before serving sprinkle with parsley or additional seasonings. For extra visual appeal and to taste brown a few extra pine nuts and sprinkle over finished dish.

Steak with Fried Leeks

1 leek, cut open, cleaned and sliced, the tough outer part
    removed
1 or 2 organic or grass-fed steaks
contents OregaMax capsules, as desired

In a frying pan heat extra virgin olive oil or coconut oil (or butter); cook leeks for about three minutes. Add steak, sprinkle contents of capsules (or use herbed garlic salt), and cook to desired doneness.

Beef and Green Bean Stew

2 lbs. beef (or lamb) roast (cut in cubes)
3 cloves garlic, sliced
contents 4 OregaMax capsules (optional)
1 teaspoon ground coriander
1 large onion, diced
1/4 cup extra virgin olive oil
2 teaspoons sea salt
3 lb. fresh or frozen green beans
1/2 teaspoon freshly ground black pepper
1 can organic tomato sauce
8 fresh tomatoes (or 1 large can whole tomatoes)

Wash and cut beans into pieces, being sure to remove stems. In a six quart pot add olive oil and heat for a minute. On medium heat add meat and spices; brown for ten minutes or so, then add onions and garlic; stir for two or three minutes. Add tomatoes and, if canned, reserve juice. Continue stirring for two more minutes. Add tomato sauce and reserved juice as well as green beans. Cook until beans are tender.

Note: if using frozen green beans, cook sauce on medium heat for a half hour before adding.

Wild Salmon with Special Vegetables & Hot Mustard

Mustard is good for the heart, because it helps open up tightened blood vessels. Plus, it is a top source of magnesium, which is desperately needed by the heart and arteries.

1 lb. wild Alaskan or Atlantic salmon
2-3 tablespoons butter or extra virgin olive oil
1 cup sliced parsnips or parsley root
1 cup leek, finely diced

1/2 cup broccoli
1/2 cup cauliflower
1 cup fish or organic chicken stock
sea salt
1/3 cup all-natural brown mustard
salt
garlic powder

In a large saucepan or skillet melt butter or use olive oil. Scatter half the vegetables in pan and cook on medium to medium low heat. Sprinkle with salt and garlic powder. Place salmon fillets in the pan besides vegetables, and add remaining vegetables. Slowly pour in fish stock. Cover and let simmer for 5 to 6 minutes only. Remove from heat. In a small saucepan add 2 tablespoons butter and melt. Add mustard and cook until hot. Serve over fish or as a dip for fish and vegetables.

Healthy Wild Salmon Salad

One large wild salmon
2 tablespoons capers
8 radishes, sliced
3 droppersful wild greens drops (i. e. GreensFlush, optional,
   to flush out any toxins)
1/2 green pepper, diced
1 medium red onion, diced
2 medium-sized organic carrots, diced
1 parsnip or parsley root, diced
vinegar to taste
extra virgin olive oil to taste
Pumpkinol (crude fortified pumpkinseed oil) to taste

In a bowl add salmon, including juice plus chopped vegetables. Drizzle with vinegar and oil to taste: note large amounts of oil give this a richer taste. Bake fish and vegetables in a 325° oven until fishi is flaky. Try to add the GreensFlush. This is important, since these greens help purge mercury. Tests show that fish eaters have much higher blood levels of this poisonous metal than non-eaters. Order GreensFlush at 1-800-243-5242.

Simple Sardine Salad

one or two cans sardines in olive oil or mustard sauce
extra virgin olive oil
balsamic vinegar
1 tablespoon diced fresh onion
3 tablespoons diced green onion tips (optional)
2 cups shredded or chopped romaine lettuce
three radishes, diced

Toss salad ingredients and top with sardines. Drizzle with olive oil and vinegar.

Simple Sardine Chopped Salad

2 parsley root or parsnips
2 carrots
1/2 cup cherry tomatoes
1 medium turnip
1/2 medium red onion
balsamic or apple cider vinegar
one or two cans sardines in water
extra virgin olive oil
Pumpkinol (crude unprocessed/fortified pumpkinseed oil)

Chop vegetables; slice tomatoes in halves. Top with sardines and drizzle liberally with olive oil, Pumpkinol, and vinegar. Serve immediately or chilled.

Buttered Wild Shrimp

8 wild shrimps (with their shells)
1 cup water
sea salt
3 slices onion
three chunks carrot
pinch fresh oregano or thyme

Remove tails and set aside to go into the sauce later. Mash the remaining shells with pestle into 1/3 cup of butter. When reduced to a paste, melt it all gradually over a low fire, stirring constantly. When the butter begins to foam, strain though a fine cheesecloth into a small bowl. On medium-low heat reheat butter mixture and add onions, carrots, spices, and shrimp. Cook just until done. Serve over a bed of romaine lettuce.

Japanese Fresh Shrimp and Vegetables

8 fresh ocean shrimp, peeled and deveined
1 1/2 oz diced green onions
1 1/2 oz. diced carrots
4 oz. grated radish
4 oz. grated turnip
2 tablespoons cold-pressed sesame oil
organic soy and shoyu sauces
wild rice (pre-cooked), optional

Over medium-low heat cook shrimp with onions; turn as necessary. Add turnips and radishes. Mix unsweetened soy and shoyu sauces to taste. Serve by itself or over a bed of wild rice.

Simple Curried Chicken

1 organic chicken, cut into pieces and ready for frying

1 chopped onion
2 to 3 teaspoons curry powder
1/2 cup fresh organic cream
2 tablespoons organic tomato paste
2 tablespoons consomme
organic butter
wild rice, cooked and ready for re-heating (optional)

In a casserole brown onion in butter until golden or light brown. Add curry powder and mix well. Sauté chicken in mixture, adding more butter, if necessary. Add cream, tomato paste, and consomme. Move and turn pieces frequently and cook for 30 to 40 minutes until tender. If sauce needs more liquid, add additional cream. For a wonderful taste sprinkle with Resvital (crude red sour grape) powder. Serve over a bed of wild rice.

Simple Sardines in Salsa-Avocado Sauce

sardines in spring water
organic tomato salsa (sugar-free)
avocado
red onion, minced (optional)
balsamic vinegar
crude fortified pumpkinseed oil (Pumpkinol)

On a plate lay sardines. Top with salsa-avocado mixture. Drizzle with vinegar and oil.

Roasted Organic Chicken in Peanut Sauce

3 lbs. (about) organic chicken
2 tablespoons organic butter
salt, freshly ground pepper, and the contents of two or more
   OregaMax capsules

Peanut sauce

1 cup skinned peanuts (you may use 1/2 natural or organic crunchy peanut butter instead)

2 tablespoons clarified butter or ghee

1 medium yellow onion, minced

1 organic tomato, chopped

1 cup organic whole milk

1 teaspoon coarse sea salt

1 capsule OregaMax

Place chicken in roasting pan. Soften butter and spread over chicken (extra virgin olive oil may be used instead); season with OregaMax and pepper. Roast at 325 degrees for about two hours. Baste with juices. For the sauce add to a blender peanuts and convert to fine paste. Using a frying pan use butter or ghee and fry onions until just golden. Stir in chopped tomatoes; cook for five to six minutes. Add peanut paste and blend well. Stir in whole milk, OregaMax, and salt. Cover and allow to simmer 20 to 30 minutes. Stir occasionally.

Unbelievable Kenyan Lamb Stew

Lamb is a heart-healthy food. This is because it is a rich source of natural fatty acids used by the heart as fuel. What's more, it contains a key nutrient required by the heart and arteries: carnitine. It is the latter which controls the entry of fuel into these organs. As the name implies, that is *carni* from carnivore, this substance is found only in animal foods. With modifications this recipe derives from the book, *Taste of Kenya* by Kathy Eldon.

1 tablespoon extra virgin olive oil

4 tablespoons ghee or organic clarified butter

2 onions, sliced

3 cloves garlic, minced
1 1/2 cups organic cherry tomatoes, cut in half
2 teaspoons fresh ginger, chopped
1 tablespoon finely chopped chilies
1/2 lb. pumpkin, peeled and cubed
3/4 cup water
1/2 teaspoon diced garlic
1 1/2 lbs. cubed lamb (from shoulder or rump)
salt and pepper
contents of three OregaMax capsules

In a thick saucepan melt 2 tablespoons ghee (this is preferable to butter, but if unavailable the latter will do); add the olive oil. Add lamb cubes seasoned with salt and pepper and brown. Remove and keep warm. In remaining oil/ghee add onions, garlic, ginger, chilies, and tomatoes and sauté for about 7 minutes. Stir in lamb and pumpkin. Cook for 25 minutes, stirring occasionally to keep from over-cooking. Pour on water, cover and cook for 40 minutes or until done and pumpkin becomes pureed. Season to taste and serve. May be served over wild rice or plain.

Sour Organic Chicken Stir-Fry

1 lb. organic chicken cut into chunks
1 head broccoli, diced
red sweet pepper, cored, minced
2 T. pomegranate syrup
3 T. extra virgin olive oil
pre-cooked wild rice (optional)
salt and pepper to taste

In a saucepan on medium heat, heat oil and brown chicken; add spices. Continue cooking until nearly done. Add broccoli, red pepper, and pomegranate syrup. Cook until vegetables are just done (noted by the bright change in color). Serve hot over bed of wild rice or plain in a bowl.

Salads

Pumpkinol-Dressed Chopped Salad

2 medium turnips, peeled and chopped into bite-sized chunks
4 organic carrots, chopped into bite-sized chunks
2 parsley root or parsnips chopped into bite-sized chunks
8 organic cherry tomatoes
3 tablespoons crude fortified pumpkinseed oil
3 tablespoons balsamic vinegar
sea salt to taste

Add all ingredients in mixing bowl; serve chilled topped with a bit of fresh parsley, dill, and or grated green zucchini.

Papaya Sprouts Salad with Avocado

organic or non-Hawaiian papaya, peeled, seeds removed (and set aside), and sliced
2 cups sprouts of your choice
1 avocado, peeled and cut in strips
1/3 red onion, cut in rings

Line avocados and papaya in a circle; top with sprouts and onion rings and chill.

Dressing
1 tablespoon papaya seeds
1/4 cup extra virgin olive oil

1/4 cup raw apple cider or balsamic vinegar
pine nuts (a few)
1 teaspoon Resvital powder (optional)
1 or 2 cloves garlic, minced
1 tablespoon or two finely minced red onion

In a blender blend until well mixed. Serve over chilled salad.

Papaya 'n Kiwi Arugula Salad

2 cups organic arugula
1 cup papaya, cut in chunks; save seeds
1 medium organic kiwi, peeled and cut in chunks
1 tablespoon pomegranate molasses
1 tablespoon lime juice
4 tablespoons extra virgin olive oil
2 tablespoons raw apple cider or balsamic vinegar

Salad dressing: in a blender add papaya seeds, clove of garlic, tablespoon pomegranate molasses, tablespoon lime juice, 4 tablespoons extra virgin olive oil, and 2 tablespoons apple cider or balsamic vinegar; blend until well mixed. Chill salad and then pour on dressing and serve.

Enzyme-Rich Fruit and Cottage Cheese Delight

large container full-fat organic cottage cheese
fresh pineapple cut into chunks (about 1/3 cup)
one kiwi fruit (select only hard fruit), peeled and diced
organic papaya (be especially careful here; the Hawaiian varieties are genetically engineered), peeled, seeded, and diced (use only about 1/4th of total, reserve the remainder)

Mix all ingredients and eat as a heart-healthy snack or as a full breakfast.

Diced Enzyme-Rich Fruit Salad

1/2 c. star fruit, diced
1/2 c. fresh pineapple, diced
1/2 c. kiwi fruit (select only hard fruit), peeled and diced
small organic papaya (be especially careful here; the Hawaiian
   varieties are genetically engineered), peeled, seeded, and diced
handful organic pecans or walnuts

Mix fruit and nuts gently. Top with freshly whipped organic
whipping cream, if desired.

Mediterranean Tomato Salad

1 1/2 lb. fresh organic tomatoes
1 medium mild red or mild yellow onion
sea salt to taste
freshly ground pepper to taste
contents 2 OregaMax capsules
2 tablespoons freshly minced parsley

Slice tomatoes and onion. In a bowl mix all ingredients and top
with Simple Middle Eastern Dressing. Or, arrange tomatoes and
onions alternately and top with all ingredients.

Famous Turkish Cucumber and Yogurt Salad

The combination of cucumber and yogurt gives great strength
to the heart and arteries, especially during the summer. This is
the ideal salad for preventing heat exhaustion. Have this before
embarking on a hot summer day.

2 medium cucumbers, peeled and diced
sea salt to taste
3 cloves raw garlic

3/4 pint whole fat organic yogurt
contents 2 OregaMax capsules
1 tablespoon crushed dried mint or 3 tablespoons chopped fresh
   mint (or use your taste to decide--add more, if desired)

Salt cucumber as desired. Leave to drain. Crush garlic with some salt. Mix in some yogurt, then add this to the remaining yogurt; mix well. Add additional salt to taste; this gives it its famous Mediterranean bite. Then, add mint and, if desired, contents of OregaMax capsules. Add drained cucumbers and mix well. May garnish with fresh mint.

Wild Rice and Nut Salad

2 cups cooked wild rice
1/4 cup whole organic pecans
2 tablespoons dried currants
half organic red sweet pepper, diced
half medium red onion, diced
1/4 cup crude fortified pumpkinseed oil (Pumpkinol)
a few tablespoons high quality balsamic vinegar
garlic salt to taste or contents of 3 OregaMax capsules

In a bowl mix all ingredients. Serve chilled, adding more vinegar, if desired.

Healthy Wild Tuna Salad

2 cans yellow fin tuna, retain juice
1 medium red sweet pepper, diced
1 medium green pepper, diced
1 medium turnip, diced
3 tablespoons capers
1/3 to 1/2 cup home-made mayonnaise

1 medium red onion, minced
8 green olives, diced
1 teaspoon wild greens drops (i.e. GreensFlush)
extra virgin olive oil
apple cider vinegar

In a bowl mix all ingredients. Drizzle with olive oil and vinegar, if desired. Makes a great dip or spread.

Beetroot and Olive Salad

Beetroot, known by Americans as simply beets (the former is the British rendition) helps detoxify the liver. So does extra virgin olive oil. A healthy liver is needed to keep the circulatory system healthy.

2 tablespoons fresh-squeezed lemon juice
2 tablespoons extra virgin olive oil
1/2 pint whole milk organic yogurt
1/2 lb. organic boiled beets, diced or sliced
2 tablespoons finely chopped parsley
flesh of 8 Greek olives, minced
sea salt to taste

In a bowl mix all ingredients. Serve chilled.

Olive oil-Enriched Spinach and Yogurt Salad

Spinach is highly nutrient dense. So is yogurt. This makes an exceptionally nutritious combination. This salad is ideal for heart and arterial health.

1 lb. fresh organic spinach
1/2 pint whole organic yogurt

1 clove garlic, crushed
2 or more tablespoons extra virgin olive oil
sea salt to taste

Wash spinach thoroughly; blend garlic with yogurt, salt, and olive oil; gently mix in spinach and serve chilled.

Soups

Old-Fashioned Mulligatawny Soup

4 yellow onions
4 tart organic apples
1 carrot
2 turnips
1/2 pound organic sirloin
4 cloves
bay leaves (or two drops of oil of bay leaf)
bunch of parsley
3 tablespoons curry powder
1 tablespoon curry paste
1/4 lb. organic butter
4 tablespoonsful organic oat or rice flour
contents five OregaMax capsules
6 quarts organic chicken or turkey broth
2 tablespoons pomegranate syrup (optional)

Cut all into slices and put into stewpan with 1/4 lb. organic butter; cook for 20 minutes on medium-low heat; then add a pint of organic chicken and turkey broth, let simmer about 20 minutes, then add curry powder, OregaMax, curry paste, and flour. Mix well together with 6 quarts of broth; when boiling, skim top. Season with salt to desired taste. For a sour taste add a tablespoon Pomegranate Syrup.

Middle Eastern Spinach and Yogurt Soup

1 lb. fresh organic spinach or 1/2 lb. frozen
1 red onion, diced
2 tablespoons extra virgin olive oil
1/4 lb. wild rice, cooked but still firm
3/4 pint whole organic yogurt
sea salt and pepper
4 organic green onions, minced
2 cloves garlic, crushed

Wash spinach leaves thoroughly; soak if necessary in water to remove all dirt. Drain and cut into large pieces or strips; do not chop. In a large saucepan heat oil; sauté onion; add spinach, stir, and cook gently. Add green onions. Cover together with wild rice. (Cover with water-about a quart) and season with salt and pepper. Bring to boil and simmer for 15 minutes. Do not allow the rice to get too mushy. Beat together yogurt and garlic. When the remainder is ready, add and mix well. Heat but do not allow the soup to boil again, or it will curdle. For additional sour taste top with Pomegranate Syrup if desired.

Extra-Ordinary Beef 'n Vegetable Broth Soup

6 quarts water
4 lbs. lean beef (for soup)
2 whole organic chickens (stewing chickens)
3 carrots
2 medium turnips
2 yellow onions

2 leeks
various fresh herbs and spices of your choice
sea salt, pepper, bay leaves as desired

In a large pot let all ingredients simmer slowly for 8 hours or until reduced to two quarts; be sure to skim and strain. Makes a large amount of soup; excess may be frozen for later use. When serving, top with chopped parsley or any fresh herb of your choice. A fantastically rich soup, ideal for heart health.

Cold Creamy Squash and Onion Soup

Squash is an ideal food for the heart and arteries. It is a rich source of vitamin A, that is as beta carotene, plus it is high in potassium. Onions help thin the blood and are a good source of vitamin C. The organic cream provides fatty compounds, needed by the heart and arteries as fuel.

1 medium to large long yellow summer squash
2 medium size yellow onions
3 tablespoons organic butter
1 cup organic cream
1/2 can organic chicken or turkey broth
1/8 teaspoon paprika
dash cinnamon

Peel squash and onions and mince finely or chop in a food processor. In a saucepan heat butter and simmer onions until clear but not brown. Add broth and squash to onion and cook until tender. Sieve and check seasoning, adding salt, pepper, and more paprika or cinnamon, if desired. Cool, add cream, and chill before serving. Garnish with freshly chopped parsley.

Purée of Turnip Soup

Turnips are a potent medicine for the heart and arteries. A rich source of heart-nourishing selenium, turnips help ward off degenerative changes in the internal organs. The regular intake of this vegetable is one of the most reliable defenses against heart and arterial disease.

4 medium turnips
1 medium onion, peeled
3 T. organic butter
1/2 c. organic cream
1/2 teaspoon freshly ground pepper
1 teaspoon coarse sea salt
8 to 12 oz. vegetable or organic chicken broth

Peel and chop turnips and onion coarsely (may use food processor). In a saucepan sauté turnips and onions in butter just until tender. Add broth and heat until bubbly. Reduce heat and add cream and seasonings and serve immediately. Note: do not salt turnips; they lose their sweet flavor and they will taste bitter. Garnish with chopped parsley or cilantro. It may be further pureed before serving.

Eggs

People with heart and arterial problems worry about eating eggs. There is nothing to worry about, that is if the eggs are natural-source. In other words, if the eggs are from truly vegetation-fed chickens, the so-called free range or organic chickens, they are safe. The fact is eggs are super-rich in nutrients, far richer than the typical foods consumed by heart or arterial disease patients. Eggs are good for the heart and arteries, because they provide nourishment, in the form of amino acids, fatty acids, vitamins, minerals, and, yes, cholesterol, which these organs desperately need to stay well. Try these egg recipes, and watch your blood pressure and heart troubles disappear.

Eggs Over-Easy with Spices

dash or two cumin powder
a few dashes coriander powder
contents of 2 OregaMax capsules
dash or two cayenne pepper
3 tablespoons extra virgin olive oil or organic butter
2 or 3 extra-large eggs
a few sprigs of parsley (washed), some minced and some whole
(about a half teaspoon minced)

In a skillet heat olive oil or butter (for frying clarified butter is ideal, but be sure it is organic). Crack eggs and gently drop into skillet. When cooked slightly sprinkle with spices. When firm, turn and sprinkle again. Salt to taste and sprinkle with parsley. Serve with sprigs of parsley; be sure to eat the sprigs.

Mediterranean Omelet

3 to 4 eggs, whipped (add full fat yogurt, if desired)
2 green onions, diced
contents of 3 to 4 OregaMax capsules
1 clove garlic, crushed
1/4 cup extra virgin olive oil

In a skillet heat oil on medium-low heat. Add garlic and onions; cook until browned. Add eggs and OregaMax contents and continue cooking, but do not over cook, as this reduces the nutritional value. Salt to taste.

Mediterranean Fried Eggs

This derives from a recipe book from the 12th century by the Middle Age Islaamic scholar, al-Baghdadi. It demonstrates a great level of advancement for such an early era.

6 organic eggs
2 to 3 tablespoons extra virgin olive oil and/or sesame oil
1 stalk celery, diced
pinch coriander, cumin, cinnamon
sea salt and freshly ground black pepper
3 tablespoons wine or apple cider vinegar

In a saucepan heat oil; add celery, a bit of finely powdered coriander, cumin, and cinnamon, then pour in vinegar plus saffron or turmeric to color. When oil is plenty hot crack eggs and add whole. When eggs set, turn off heat and pour oil back over yolks to set further and serve.

Egg 'n Onion Souffle

1 medium finely minced yellow onion
4 organic/free range eggs
1 clove garlic, crushed
5 tablespoons organic butter
2 tablespoons whole wheat or whole oat flour
salt and pepper to taste
1 cup organic chicken stock
1 teaspoon parsley, finely minced
dash cayenne pepper

In a saucepan melt butter and add onions, stirring over moderate heat until onion is soft. Add flour and stir well. Pour in stock and cook until sauce is smooth, stirring to prevent any sticking.

Add spices but not parsley. In a bowl beat eggs, the yolks and whites separately. Add the yolks first, then fold in whites lightly into the whole. Pour into an ungreased casserole placed in a pan of water, add parsley, and bake in a preheated oven at 350 degrees. To check doneness use a stainless silver knife until it comes out clean (about a half hour or a little more).

Cereals and Dessert

Oat Bran Cereal

This is the only cereal allowed on this plan. The fact is oat bran is an ideal food for the heart and arteries. It is significantly richer in B-vitamins than oatmeal. Plus, it is lower in starch. Oat bran is a top source of B-vitamins as well as selenium, silicon, and magnesium and it is also a good source of iron and phosphorus. The Nutri-Sense fortifies it even further, since it is a top source of niacin and thiamine.

water
salt
oat bran cereal (follow directions on box)
2 tablespoons Nutri-Sense
cinnamon
wild raw honey, i. e. wild oregano, dandelion, or thistle honey

Cook oat bran cereal according to instructions. Serve hot topped with Nutri-Sense, cinnamon, and wild honey.

Honey-Nut Wild Berry Dessert

This is your main dessert, that is any combination of nuts and wild berries. The availability of wild berries is limited, that is unless you pick your own. A crude raw honey is acceptable, that is if it is truly crude, raw, and from bees not fed sugar. Another option is the same dessert with frozen organic strawberries instead of blueberries. However, in major health food store chains, such as Whole Foods and Wild Oats, wild blueberries are available. They may also be available in specialty stores and gourmet grocery stores.

wild blueberries
wild oregano or thistle honey
pine nuts (these are usually wild)
wild hickory nuts (use pecans as an alternative)
walnuts

Mix together and drizzle with raw wild honey.
Note: to order truly wild and non-sugar fed bee honey call 1-800-243-5242.

Honey-Nut, Version #2

wild blueberries
organic strawberries
raw organic almonds
raw organic pecans
raw organic sunflower seeds

Mix together all ingredients and drizzle with raw wild honey. As an alternative add all ingredients in bowl of organic half 'n half and drizzle with honey.

Sauces, Dressings, and More

Simple Middle Eastern Salad Dressing

1 or 2 tablespoons fresh lemon juice

3 tablespoons extra virgin olive oil
1 clove garlic, crushed
sea salt and freshly ground black pepper
minced parley

Blend all ingredients and use fresh on any salad.

Old Fashioned French Tomato Sauce

1 can cooked organic tomatoes
1 small can organic tomato paste
1 medium onion, chopped
pinch each of chopped thyme and parsley
pinch salt and 1/4 tsp freshly ground black pepper
1 bay leaf

Boil down to proper consistency and strain. Refrigerate for future use.

Vintage (1940s) French Dressing

This is the kind of French dressing that existed before the food processors corrupted it. It is free of all the obnoxious ingredients found in the commercial versions. This is French dressing as it was originally prepared.

2/3 teaspoon coarse sea salt
black peppercorns, about 6
1 tablespoon red wine vinegar
3 1/2 tablespoons extra virgin olive oil

Grind the peppercorns and sea salt in a mill. Mix all ingredients together. Whip until thickened. Toss into salad. This dressing is ideal for bibb lettuce and/or watercress.

Home-Made All-Natural Mayonnaise

I have adapted this from a combination of the recipes in Martha Stewart's superb book, *Hors d'Oeuvres* and my own version in *How to Eat Right and Live Longer*.

2 eggs
1/4 teaspoon dry mustard
dash cayenne pepper
1/2 teaspoon coarse sea salt
2 tablespoons apple cider vinegar
1 cup extra virgin olive oil
1 cup cold-pressed hazelnut, walnut, or sunflower oil

In the bowl of a food processor or blender put eggs, mustard, cayenne, sea salt, and vinegar. Combine the oils and begin processing, adding the oil only a drop at a time, that is until mixture thickens. Add the rest of the oil in a steady stream. Refrigerate immediately and serve chilled. As an alternative add finely minced herbs in the initial mix.

Sesame Seed Paste Surprise

Sesame seeds contain a substance which prevents, even reverses, arterial disease. This is known as sesamol, one of the most potent antioxidants known.

2 medium garlic cloves
sea salt to taste
juice of 3 organic lemons or limes
1/2 pint sesame seed (tahini) paste
1/2 teaspoon cumin
contents 2 OregaMax capsules (optional)
7 tablespoons parsley, finely minced

1 teaspoon Sesam-E
pomegranate fruit (i. e. a few fruit seeds)

In a firm bowl crush garlic with salt. Add sesame seed paste; mix. Add lemon juice until fully mixed; dilute with cold water to improve consistency. Season with more salt plus cumin; top with Sesam-E, pomegranate seeds, and the contents of OregaMax capsules, if desired. Before serving cover each serving with chopped parsley.

Sesame Seed Paste-Plus (with walnuts)

Both walnuts and sesame seeds help nourish the heart and arteries. Studies prove that the regular intake of these nuts/seeds helps prevent circulatory diseases. This recipe is adapted from Claudia Roden's *Book of Middle Eastern Food.*

1/2 lb. organic walnuts
3 tablespoons sesame seed paste
a few sesame seeds
sea salt
2 cloves garlic
juice of 2 medium lemons
5 tablespoons minced parsley
1 teaspoon oil of Sesam-E

Pound walnuts and garlic in mortar or strong bowl with a bit of salt, that is until walnuts are nearly a paste. Add sesame seed paste and lemon juice little by little, stirring thoroughly. Next, mix in parsley. This may also be done in a blender, by adding lemon juice and sesame seed paste slowly along with walnuts and garlic; blend thoroughly without over-blending walnuts. Add water to desired thickness. Top with Sesam-E and parsley. Great as a dip for vegetables.

Vegetable Dishes

Mashed turnips

organic turnips
sea salt

Boil turnips until extremely soft (must be soft enough to pass through a sieve). The pulp is then placed in a cloth, which is rolled and wrung, one person at each end. The pulp is then mixed with softened butter and cream, to desired taste. Add salt and pepper, as well as garlic powder, as desired. Turnips are rich in selenium and sulfur, which greatly strengthen the heart.

Curried Vegetables

4 organic carrots, cut in chunks
2 medium organic turnips, cut in chunks
2 red onions, diced
2 stalks celery, diced
1 medium organic red sweet pepper, diced
1 cup whole organic milk
1/4 pound organic butter
curry powder (to taste)
curry paste (to taste)
extra organic butter or spiced coconut oil (i.e. CocaPalm)
wild rice
sea salt

Cook vegetables in butter or spiced coconut oil (i. e. CocaPalm), sprinkling with curry powder to let them absorb it. Stir in curry paste, simmer the vegetables until tender. Add milk and also more butter or coconut oil as needed. Prepare wild rice by boiling in salt water until just tender and separate vegetables and rice in a divided dish. The vegetables must absorb all the sauce in which they are simmered. The more curry powder that is used the better it is for the heart and arteries.

Ghee-Fried Carrots

the upper round parts of 14 or more carrots
ghee or a spiced coconut oil (i.e. CocaPalm)

Cut the upper part of 14 carrots, that is the round thinner portion, leaving the rest for salads, etc. Blanch these rounds. In a deep frying pan heat ghee or CocaPalm. Fry as potatoes until done.

Yogurt-Eggplant Purée

This is a tasty and nourishing dish, ideal for promoting healthy arteries. The full-fat yogurt provides the fatty acids needed for nourishing the heart and arterial muscles.

3 eggplants
4 tablespoons extra virgin olive oil
1/2 pint full-fat organic yogurt
juice of one lemon or lime
2 medium garlic cloves, crushed
sea salt
3 tablespoons finely minced parsley

Grill eggplants, preferably over charcoal, which creates the distinctive roasted flavor. They may also be simply grilled over an inside grill or gas flame. Scar them until skin starts to blister and turns black. Under the faucet (cold) rub off the skins; remove all charred particles. Gently squeeze out as much juice as possible, since it is bitter.

Put the eggplants in a bowl and mash with a fork, or blend them in a blender. Add the oil, little by little, beating or blending continuously. Then, add yogurt and mix vigorously, until it is thoroughly mixed within the puree. Mix in remaining ingredients, holding back parsley; spoon into a bowl and garnish with parsley. Serve cold.

Fried Eggplant with Yogurt

3 medium eggplants
sea salt
extra virgin olive oil
3 cloves garlic, crushed
teaspoon red sour grape powder (Resvital powder), optional
1/2 pint full-fat organic yogurt
teaspoon dried crushed mint

Wash outside and cut eggplants into large slices, about 1/2 inch thick. Salt and leave in colander for about 1/2 hour to allow bitter juices to drain. Rinse with cold water; let drain/dry.

Heat extra virgin olive oil; add a few drops oil of wild rosemary or oregano to prevent toxicity; cook until eggplant is slightly browned on each side. Add garlic and continue browning for a few moments; remove to dish or brown paper towels (for absorbing excess fat); allow to cool. Now add yogurt and salt, layering the eggplant on a dish. Garnish with red sour grape powder and dried mint or parsley. Highly nourishing.

Simple Sour Onion Salad

2 large red onions
3 to 4 tablespoons apple cider or wine vinegar
teaspoon Resvital (red sour grape) powder (optional but medicinal)

teaspoon chopped fresh mint or parsley

Slice or dice onions. In a mixing bowl add onions and all other ingredients; gently toss until mixed. Serve as a side dish with any meat or vegetable entree.

Cucumbers with Dill and Sour Cream

Cucumbers are good for the heart. They have a mild diuretic action. Cucumbers help the body retain healthy fluids, while washing out toxins.

3 medium-sized cucumbers, peeled and diced
1 cup organic sour cream
sea salt
1 tablespoon apple cider vinegar
3 tablespoons fresh chopped dill
1 tablespoon fresh lemon juice

In a bowl combine salt, lemon juice, vinegar, and dill with sour cream and mix. Add cucumber. Serve chilled and garnish with additional dill.

Artichoke Hearts in Heavy Oil

Artichoke hearts are good for the heart. This vegetable contains inulin, which helps strengthen all organs, particularly the liver and pancreas. Artichokes are also a good source of folic acid, needed for healthy heart and arteries.

can artichoke hearts (about 14 -to 16- ounces)
1/3 cup extra virgin olive oil
juice of 2 lemons
teaspoon Resvital powder (optional)

2 cloves garlic
sea salt

Drain artichokes thoroughly. In a skillet heat olive oil and garlic; add artichokes, lemon juice, Resvital, and salt; simmer for 10 to 15 minutes.

Beverages

Pomegranate Surprise

Pomegranate has been recently shown to be beneficial to the heart and arteries. This fruit contains a flavonoid, which helps prevent stickiness of the blood. This is one of the most heart-healthy drinks possible. Pomegranate Syrup is made by Super-Market Remedies, 1-800-243-5242.

Pomegranate Syrup
sparkling mineral water
ice

In a lemonade pitcher mix four ounces Pomegranate Syrup with two quarts sparkling water; beware of the fizz; mix slowly. Add sprigs of mint and ice, if desired. Serve chilled or on ice.

WildPower Tea

This tea is ideal for circulatory disorders, because it is a natural diuretic. What's more, it is completely safe, even for use with medication. The ingredients are wild strawberry leaves, wild hibiscus flowers, and wild borage flowers. Again, this is completely safe for all ages and for anyone taking medication. In fact, it reduces the need for drugs.

five or more tablespoons WildPower Tea
purified (chlorine-free) water

Boil a quart of water. While boiling add the tea. Turn off heat, cover and let steep, preferably overnight. Reheat or serve chilled. Add raw honey and cream, if desired.

Note: this is a natural but gentle diuretic. In a waterlogged person, it may cause weight loss. WildPower Tea is available from North American Herb & Spice.

Wild Labrador Leaf Brew

12 oz. bottle wild brew (labrador tea leaves plus wild rose hips, pre-brewed)
spring water

In a tea pot add one part wild brew to two parts spring water. Heat and serve; add a teaspoon of raw honey and/or whole organic milk, if desired. This is an excellent way to consume on a daily basis fresh natural vitamin C plus wild-source aromatic compounds. For thousands of years labrador leaves have been brewed by Native Americans to make an immune-enhancing tea. Note: this wild brew is available from North American Herb & Spice.

Note: for all recipes: when cooking with oil and butter, always sauté at the lowest temperature.

Conclusion

Infection plays a primary role in circulatory disease. Medical textbooks confirm that a wide range of disorders of the heart and arteries are due to infection. Inflammation of the arteries, hardening of the arteries, arterial scarring, heart valve disorders, congestive heart failure, enlarged heart syndrome (cardiomyopathy), and high blood pressure, all have proven infectious causes. There are entire categories of heart disease fully due to infection, for instance, endocarditis and cardiomyopathy. Despite this the role of infection in circulatory diseases is little known in the medical profession, nor are the victims of these diseases usually aware of it. People continue with their medical therapies—drugs and invasive procedures— while having no clue that their problem is largely infective. The fact is in many instances the drugs and invasive procedures deepen the infection, increasing the risks for sudden death.

How great of a role infection plays varies with each individual. Suffice it to say that if there exists a chronic infection there is no means to cure this disease, that is unless the infection is eradicated. The complete eradication of such infections results in complete—and permanent—cures. Imagine: heart disease and/or high blood pressure, cured. This would be a landmark in scientific and humanitarian achievement. The fact is this can readily be accomplished, merely by eradicating any sites of infection. As early as the 1930s Price, as well as Fischer, documented the reversal of heart disease: by curing the causative infections.

The fact is if the underlying infection is destroyed overall health will improve. This includes the health of all organs, including the cardiovascular system. It must improve and it must do so relatively quickly, because the burden has been relieved, the inflammation halted, and the infection obliterated.

Spice oils, particularly oil of wild oregano, are potent germicides. Plus, they are safe for internal use, far safer than common alternatives such as hydrogen peroxide, antibiotics, and iodine. Regarding the former this usually causes recession of the gums. Regarding iodine there is always a risk for allergic reactions. What's more, both these substances are synthetic chemicals: the oil of wild oregano, that is the Oreganol P73, is purely natural.

The Oreganol is a product of nature. Truly, it is divine in source. No human invented it. The fact is it is the natural medicine par excellence. What's more, the true wild oregano, the Oreganol P73, is the natural spice oil, fully edible. This is while causing no harm it helps reverse disease. The same is true of the other truly edible spice oils mentioned in this book.

Consider that chemical antiseptics, that is chlorinated compounds, hydrogen peroxide, and iodine, are synthetic chemicals, produced in laboratories. There is no comparison between these and the oil of wild oregano. The fact is the wild oregano oil reigns supreme. What's more, this entire program is based upon unprocessed natural medicines that cannot be duplicated by synthetic medicines. Nor can dentistry offer any similar alternatives.

Only nature can cure. This is certainly the case with the wild oregano, that is as a means to purge infection and to eradicate any hidden site of germs. It is also the case with crude sour grape, natural fruit enzymes, and the other highly potent natural medicines mentioned herein. These safe and effective natural medicines are wild spice extracts for killing germs, particularly the oils of edible wild oregano and clove buds (or for dental purposes, the OregaDENT).

There is also the crude red sour grape for regenerating the arterial wall, oil of garlic/onion, for cleansing the arteries, lymph, and blood, while providing a natural source of energizing sulfur, fruit-source enzymes, which open up constrictions and blockages. Wild berry and greens extracts act as general cleansers and natural diuretics. Wild strawberry and blueberry leaf-based teas are natural diuretics. What's more, raw wild honey, particularly the wild oregano honey, improves digestion, while purging excess fluids and nourishing the tissues. Potent fruit-source enzymes, for instance, the Infla-eez, dissolve clots as well as plaque. This leads to a dramatic improvement in blood flow.

The oregano should always be taken with plant flavonoids, especially grape flavonoids. Such flavonoids are found in rich amounts in the village formula, Resvital. It is the Resvital, which helps improve the elasticity of the arterial walls, a crucial element of the high blood pressure cure. Thus, the wild oregano products plus the Resvital make an ideal treatment system. Other supplements help speed the cure: oil of cold-pressed garlic, fruit enzymes, and diuretic agents such as wild cranberry and wild berry leaf tea. All such substances are listed in Appendix A. This is a natural protocol free of side effects. The ideal oregano to take is the OregaBiotic, although some people prefer to use the oregano oil. Such formulas are crucial, since it is the spice oils which purge dangerous germs from the heart and arteries.

Regarding supplements only the purest most high-grade sources must be used. For such medicines, in fact, foods, to be effective they must be carefully processed to avoid alteration or corruption. It is only the truly natural substances, as unaltered as possible, which create cures. This demonstrates the value of the divine source in human benefit: drugs fail to cure, while natural substances achieve this. North American Herb & Spice provides truly natural substances, unaltered by man and created by almighty God.

This is far from an attempt to preach. It is merely a fact of chemistry. The natural substances help reverse disease, while the synthetic chemicals cause disease. The latest pharmaceutical catastrophes, Vioxx, Bextra, Celebrex, Aleve, Baycol, Fen-Fen, and countless others, prove that.

Few people realize how powerful the unaltered natural substances are. They have a trapped energy, that of harnessed sunlight. It is a photonic energy never found in synthetic drugs. Only this power is capable of healing. Only this source can reverse the degenerative diseases, which afflict humankind.

There is a power in this universe. It can be sensed. One way to harness this is to use the mightily powered natural cures. This means that synthetic or 'dead' drugs must be avoided. By taking the truly unaltered cures a revolution can occur: in the individual's personal health. Such natural cures are capable of reversing virtually any disease, including high blood pressure. Seemingly, virtually any disease can be reversed by such substances. Take advantage of the power of these substances. Regardless of your condition your health will dramatically improve as a result.

Appendix

Numerous chemicals, as well as processed foods, can damage the heart. What's more, the arteries and veins are also readily poisoned by synthetic chemicals, particularly drugs and food additives. Genetically engineered substances, which have contaminated the food, also poison the critical organs. The fact is sudden death is a consequence of the consumption of such foods. These chemicals are synthetic: man-made poisons, which destroy the cells and organs. Such chemicals weaken the body, increasing the risks for a variety of diseases.

Every effort should be made to read labels and understand the true nature of a given 'food', that is before purchasing. The food processors have only one interest: corporate profits. It is up to the individual to take responsibility for his/her health. If you fail to take care of yourself, who will? Each person is on his or her own. So, read labels. Know what the food is before you buy it. Use your buying power to protest against food toxins: if the food or beverage contains any of the following toxins, do not buy it. Only through such an approach can change occur.

Only then will the perpetrators of these crimes come forward and change their destructive ways. If you care about your body, do not knowingly feed it harsh poisons.

Foods toxic to the heart and arteries

In order for the high blood pressure reversal plan to work the following foods must be strictly avoided. Do not deviate. Avoid the following completely:

nitrated meats
pork products
white flour
white rice
white bread, buns, rolls, etc.
cookies, candies, cakes, pies, donuts, sweet rolls, muffins, etc.
commercial cereals containing refined grains, sugar, etc.
margarine
hydrogenated and partially hydrogenated oils
deep fried foods (unless home cooked in heart-healthy oils)
candy bars of all types
foods containing aspartame
white flour-based pastas, noodles, lasagna, etc.
foods containing white sugar or corn syrup, including commercial ketchup, relish, tomato sauces, steak sauce, salad dressing, and yogurt
sugared nuts
caramels and taffy
chocolates of any type
puddings and custard of all kinds
commercial peanut butter or foods containing it
ice cream, ice milk, sherbet, and similar sugar- and food dye-contaminated frozen desserts

By strictly avoiding such foods a noticeable reduction in blood pressure will occur. Of note sugar causes fluid retention, which aggravates the high blood pressure tendency and can play a primary role in its cause.

Beverages toxic to the heart and arteries

In order for the high blood pressure reversal plan to work the following beverages must be strictly avoided. Do not deviate. Avoid the following completely:

soda pop
iced tea
hot chocolate
chocolate milk
black tea with sugar
sweetened condensed milk
coffee
iced coffee drinks
malts
shakes
floats
Kool-Aid
fruit drinks
hard liquor
beer
wine
wine coolers
sports drinks
Slim Fast-type weight loss or nutritive drinks
Gatorade-like drinks, that is sports drinks containing sugars
instant breakfast-type drinks
malted milk

ice slushes
refined apple juice
Ovaltine, PDQ, and Nestle's Quick
lemonade (made with white sugar or corn syrup)
chlorinated water

By strictly avoiding such beverages a noticeable reduction in blood pressure will usually occur.

Foods containing hydrogenated or partially hydrogenated oils

In the supermarket there are hundreds of foods, which contain these oils. Again, recent evidence implicates hydrogenated and partially hydrogenated oils in the cause of heart and circulatory diseases, while, for instance, butter, coconut oil, and extra virgin olive oil have not been implicated. What's more, such research is proving that while butter fails to raise cholesterol levels there is a significant elevation as a result of the consumption of margarine as well as foods contaminated with margarine-like oils. To ensure a reduction or normalization of blood pressure the intake of hydrogenated and partially hydrogenated oils must be strictly prohibited. Completely avoid the following:

candy bars
salted nut rolls
hard candies
taffy, caramels, and toffee
margarine
commercial peanut butter
commercial crackers
imitation ice cream

Egg-Beaters
microwave popcorn
imitation whipping cream and non-dairy creamer
donuts and sweet rolls
fruit pies, cupcakes, Ho-Hos, Twinkies, etc.
cinnamon rolls
frozen or restaurant pizzas
breaded fish, chicken, beef, and pork
French fries and Tater Tots
tortilla chips
Cheetos, cheese puffs, and corn chips
potato chips (some)
Pringle's-Style potato chips
imitation cheese spread
egg rolls
puddings and/or pudding pops
ice cream sticks, cakes, and pops
creamed vegetables
instant mashed potatoes
toaster pastries
donuts and pastries
croissants and muffins
commercial breakfast and/or granola bars
tacos (i.e. the shells)
commercial salad dressings (some)
cocoa mix (some)

Foods containing sulfites

Sulfites can cause severe toxicity to the body, largely through the process of oxidation. That is these chemicals directly oxidize the cells, causing severe tissue damage. Sulfite may cause shock reactions, and this may result in heart spasms, arrhythmia, hypertension, even heart attacks and strokes. Food sources include:

pickle relish
pickles
white and red wine
champagne
wine coolers
vinegar
shredded coconut
dried citrus fruit-based beverage mixes
dried fruit (unless organic)
restaurant shrimp
breading and batters
canned fruit
canned vegetables (some)
cole slaw (some)
cornstarch
fish products
frozen vegetables
fruit drinks
fruit salad
fruit toppings
guacamole (some, added to preserve color)
hard candy
instant tea
jams and jellies
potato salad
relishes of all types
dried or canned soup
white and brown sugar

Foods containing MSG

MSG is a neurotoxin. Swartz notes in his book, *In Bad Taste*, that this substance is one of the most potent neurological toxins known. It clearly upon regular consumption causes brain damage. MSG is found exclusively in processed and restaurant food.

MSG is deemed by the food industry as a flavor enhancer. The fact is all it does is enhance an individual's discomfort. People get violently ill from its consumption. Typical symptoms include a tight band around the headache, as well as migraines, hives, itchy skin, diarrhea, and overall bizarre sensations. Then, there is the Chinese Restaurant Syndrome, characterized by burning sensations, chest pain, palpitations, facial pressure, headaches, heartburn, and diarrhea. Despite this the food industry claims MSG is safe. Yet, are such symptoms the sign of a safe food? The fact is no truly safe food should cause such symptoms. Even so, not all people react to it. People with weakened immune systems are particularly vulnerable. Thus, perhaps the greatest problem with MSG is allergic reactions, as demonstrated by the following:

CASE HISTORY:

Mr. B. is a respected media personality with a serious allergic tendency. He reacts strongly to MSG, which causes him to break out in hives. Normally very fastidious about his diet he was urged constantly by friends to try the cheese dip. It was the type of dip, he knew, that usually contains MSG. He ate some and within three hours broke out in itchy hives. A big fan of the wild oregano he took it with significant results. The results were, in fact, dramatic: a near complete elimination of itching and inflammation. Plus, he rubbed it on the hives, and it immediately relieved both the itching and swelling. Upon checking further he found that, in fact, the cheese dip contained MSG.

The problem isn't with the molecule, that is monosodium glutamate, per se. The ingredients of this substance are naturally occurring and are found within soybeans and seaweed. This is what gives such foods their powerful flavor. In fact, seaweed and fermented soy products are a concentrate of this molecule. In the natural state as a part of the whole food MSG is relatively harmless. It is the isolate that is of concern. Because of the vast usage of this substance it is produced synthetically. The raw materials from which the molecule is derived are primarily corn, wheat, and sugar beets, which are common allergens. Plus, regarding the corn and sugar beets these are genetically engineered, which accelerates the toxicity. Thus, for those who love the flavor of MSG there is an option to the isolated chemical: the addition of soy sauce and seaweed, the naturally occurring sources of this substance, to the food.

In particular for people with sensitive systems, as well as people with weakened immunity, MSG should be avoided. Even so, tests show that this food additive causes brain lesions in animals. Because of such research all people should avoid MSG. Due to its toxic effects upon the nervous system it must also be avoided on the hypertension cure plan. One issue is certain: MSG offers no nutritional value to food. Thus, why is it added to the food supply? It is added only to enhance corporate profits by creating an addictive taste sensation. I nearly always react to MSG; my most debilitating symptoms are digestive distress and insomnia. Thus, I avoid it like the plague. The primary sources of this substance include:

Accent or Lawry's Seasoning
bacon bits
baking mixes

batters
beef jerky
bouillon cubes
bread stuffings
breaded deep fried foods
breaded frozen foods
breading
brown or cream gravies and sauces
canned meats
canned tuna (certain brands)
cheese dips and sauces
cheese puffs
Chef Boyardee products
chicken and beef spreads
dry roasted mixed nuts
dry roasted cashews
dry roasted peanuts
dry roasted sunflower seeds
croutons
chip dip
Chinese food, canned
frozen dinners
frozen pizza
frozen pot pies
frozen potato products
gelatins
packed noodles or pasta
potato chips (some)
health food store chips (some)
processed meats (hot dogs, bologna, salami, bacon, etc.)
processed cheeses

processed poultry products
puddings
relishes
salad dressings
salt substitutes
seasonings
soft candies
soups, canned or instant
stew, canned

Note: MSG may also be listed on labels as hydrolyzed vegetable protein, which is about 40% MSG by weight, or even natural flavors.

Bibliography

Bateman, M. 1991. *Good Enough to Eat*. London: Sinclair-Stevenson, Ltd.

Bothwell, J. 1950. *Onions without Tears*. New York: Hastings House.

Burtis, E. L. 1960. *The Real American Tragedy*. Milwaukee, WI: Royal Lee Foundation.

Caliguiri, F. 1964. *Guide to Your Spice Shelf*. San Francisco, CA: Spice Islands.

Clark, Linda. 1976. *Linda Clark's Handbook of Natural Remedies for Common Ailments*. New York: Pocketbooks.

Cross, R. 1974. *The Honey & Yoghurt Cookbook*. London: W. Foulsham & Co., Ltd.

Duncan, G. 1959. *Diseases of Metabolism*. New York: W. B. Saunders Co.

Eldon, K. and E. Mullan. 1985. *Tastes of Kenya*. Nairobi.

Finnegan, John. 1993. *The Facts About Fats*. Berkely, CA: Celestial Arts.

Fischer, M. H. 1940. *Death and Dentistry*. Lancaster, PA: Science Press Printing Co.

Griffith, Linda and Fred. 1994. *Onions/Onions/Onions*. Shelbourne, VT: Chapter's.

Hanke, M. *Diet and Dental Health.* 1933. Chicago, IL: University of Chicago Press.

Heard, G. W. 1952. *Man vs. Toothache*. Milwaukee, WI: Lee Foundation for Nutritional Research.

Humphrey, S. W. 1965. *Spices, Seasonings, and Herbs: the Definitive Cookbook*. New York: Macmillon.

Ingram, Cass. 2004. *Nutrition Tests for Better Health.* Buffalo Grove, IL: Knowledge House.

Ingram, Cass. 2001. *How to Eat Right and Live Longer.* Buffalo Grove, IL: Knowledge House.

Ingram, Cass. 1991. *Who Needs Headaches?* Cedar Rapids, IA: Literary Visions.

Isselbacher, K. J., et al. 1980. *Harrison's Principles of Internal Medicine.* New York: McGraw-Hill.

Kato, Y. 1973. *Garlic: The Unknown Miracle Worker.* Japan: Oyama Garlic Laboratory

Pomeranz, H. and I. S. Koll. 1951. *The Family Physician*. New York: Greystone Press.

Price, J. M. 1969. *Coronaries/Cholesterol/Chlorine.* New York: Jove Publications.

Price, Weston A. 1923. *Dental Infections and the Degenerative Diseases.* Vol. II. Cleveland, OH: Penton Publ. Co.

Rees, M. K. 1988. *The Complete Guide to Living with High Blood Pressure.* Mount Vernon, NY: Consumer's Union.

Roden, C. 1968. *A Book of Middle Eastern Food.* Middlesex: Penguin.

Rorty, James and N. P. Norman. 1956. *Tomorrow's Food.* New York: Devon-Adair.

Rudolph, T. M. 1957. *Vitamin "E".* Los Angeles, CA: Nutrition Research Publ. Co.

Salinger, J. L. and F. J. Kalteyer. 1900. *Modern Medicine.* Philadelphia: W. B. Saunders & Co.

Shafer, W. G., Hine, M. K. and B. M. Levy. 1963. *Textbook of Oral Pathology.* Philadelphia: W. B. Saunders Co.

Stewart, Martha. 1984. *Hors d'Oeuvres.* New York: Clarkson N. Potter, Inc.

Tietze, H. W. *Papaya: The Healing Fruit.* Vancouver, BC: Alive Books.

von Noorden, C. 1904. *Diseases of Metabolism and Nutrition.* New York: B. B. Treat & Co.

Addendum

The Miracle of Vitamin C. Sunnivale, CA: Research Publications.

A Prescription with 5000 Years of History. Tadworth/Surrey: Allysol Co.

Index

G

H

NOTES